Anxiety Control Guide for Kids

A Simple Anxiety Relief Guide to Regulate Worry,
Fear, Insecurities and Stress

BY

Koala Publishers

Jasmine O'Brien

By reading this text, the reader accepts that the author will not be held liable for any damages, indirectly or directly, experienced due to the use of the information included herein, particularly, but not limited to, omissions, errors, or inaccuracies. As a reader, you are accountable for your decisions, actions, and consequences.

About the Author

Jasmine O' Brien is a child psychiatrist with a deep understanding of child behavior and mental illnesses. She has spent more than 8 years in the field helping tons of children suffering from anxiety, depression, chronic stress, phobias, and much more. She also has years-long experience as the parent of a child with GAD (Generalized Anxiety Disorder.) She understands the helplessness of parenting a child with anxiety and hopes to help parents like these on a broader scale with her professional expertise.

"Anxiety Control for Kids" is one of her famous marvels on parenting kids with troubled psychology and behavior, among many other educational and interactive books.

Table of contents

Introduction

Did you know? One out of every eight kids in the USA and one out of every six kids in the UK struggle with an anxiety disorder.

Anxiety is treatable. However, according to a 2015 Child Mind Institute Report, 80 percent of children with a diagnosable anxiety disorder do not receive due attention or treatment.

Is your kid one of the millions of children worldwide struggling with anxiety?

Is he receiving your due attention?

Anxiety is a common and often useful emotion too as it helps to strive for better. But when a person experiences disproportionate anxiety levels regularly, it can constitute a medical condition.

Anxiety disorders are a group of mental issues characterized by extreme uneasiness, apprehension, fear, and worry. These disorders cause physical symptoms as well as changes in how a person processes emotions and how he behaves. Mild anxiety might be vague and disturbing, whereas severe anxiety can significantly impact daily life.

Anxiety in children manifests as stomach problems, headaches, or behavioral concerns such as temper tantrums. In children, restlessness, avoidance, inattention, and frequent meltdowns are all common anxiety symptoms. Unfortunately, these symptoms are frequently misinterpreted as moodiness, laziness, and stubbornness.

Children cannot say things like "I have anxiety" or "I am very worried" because their verbal skills are still developing.

But how does your child feel on the inside?

Can you recall how it feels to be on a rollercoaster's highest point? Remember how you felt when you were on the verge of going over the edge. It is a stomach-churning feeling that lasts only a few seconds, but it can last for days or even weeks in people with chronic anxiety.

This is one of the many complex feelings of your child.

As a parent, it can be terribly overwhelming and confusing to see your child struggle with mental health issues, especially if it is something you cannot understand. As a parent, it is your responsibility to support your children. Let me be your helping hand in this journey.

The inspiration behind this book is to help you empower your children and not lose themselves to the bully in their head. The first part of the book is focused on understanding the concept of anxiety, where it comes from, and how it affects your child. You will find real-life stories of anxiety stricken kids to help you understand what your child feels. This way, you can better relate to your child and change your parenting style accordingly to relieve the problem. You will also be provided with an anxiety guide for your child before entering into the practical part of the book.

The next four chapters of this anxiety relief book offer you effective parental strategies to parent your child riddled with anxiety. This part will deal with worry, fear, insecurities, and stress one by one head-on and help you ensure a satisfying and happy life for your child.

But how do you believe I am worthy of your time and effort?

I have been a child psychiatrist for more than eight years. I provide my expertise to children with all kinds of mental illnesses, especially anxiety and depression, every day. I have had hundreds of children like your child come to me and have shown remarkable progress.

The strategies I have put together in this book come from my professional knowledge and my personal knowledge as a parent. My fourteen-year-old boy was diagnosed with GAD (Generalized Anxiety Disorder) at age 9. He is in a much better mental state now, and I feel grateful that I had the professional knowledge and experience to deal with it. I realize all parents do not have this privilege, and I see the helplessness in parents' eyes every day. Therefore, it is my goal to spread this knowledge on a broader scale.

Children get anxious. They can take everything very seriously, whether it is a fear of the dark, getting another pimple or starting a new school. However, some children are more concerned than others. It is never easy to watch a little one suffer at the hands of anxiety, but it is even more difficult when you are not sure if she is worrying excessively and needs help.

The severity of the anxiety distinguishes normal to worry from anxiety disorders. While anxiety is a normal response to stressful situations, it becomes a disorder when it intervenes with a child's ability to manage ordinary situations or causes them to avoid activities that most other children of their age enjoy.

So let's begin and guide your child towards living his life to the fullest without his worries and fears drowning him.

Chapter 1: Be in Your Child's Shoes

275 million people struggle with anxiety disorders around the globe.

Anxiety can manifest itself in various ways for these millions of people, ranging from continuous worry, overwhelm, and a whole-body clenching feeling to the paralyzed catastrophe of a full-blown panic attack. Everything feels bad, and you are always trying to get out of it, which usually makes things worse. But, it is all diagnosable, manageable, and eventually treatable.

Anxiety may feel terrible by definition, but it does not mean it is always bad. It is a harsh world, and your brain needs a mechanism to shift your attention when you are in danger. Two brain regions are responsible for this: the amygdala, which is located deep in the brain's basement, and the upper, more complex cerebral cortex.

The amygdala processes very basic emotions — fear, anger, guilt, and jealousy — and handles them rapidly and unconsciously as it befits its lowly location. The terror you feel when confronted by a threatening stranger and the fear you feel when watching a terrifying movie both trigger the same amygdala alarms and do so in less than 20 milliseconds, which is a good thing if the danger is real. The cerebral cortex is in charge of determining whether it is or is not, and it thinks the things through more calmly before responding to the threat or turning off the amygdala's alarm.

The alarm, on the other hand, might sometimes get stuck. When attempting to distinguish actual dangers from exaggerated ones, the cerebral cortex might become confused. For example, doorknobs contain germs, but how can you be sure the one you touched was not infected? People are subjected to social humiliation at parties or while giving speeches; how do you know you would not be one of them? This overly active and obsessive alarm provokes exaggerated responses in individuals with anxiety.

Now let's enter into the world of anxiety to know what you are dealing with.

1.1 Living with Anxiety

A 7-year-old is an excellent student, but he messes up his room and shouts at his siblings after school. A ten-year-old frequently snaps at her mother, criticizing everything she does. Every morning before school, an 8-year-old sobs and clings to his parents as they attempt to drop him off at school, sports events, or birthday parties. Headaches make it tough for a 12-year-old to get out of the door on time. A six-year-old is unable to sleep at night. Even though these behaviors look unrelated and pose different challenges, they all share one thing in common: anxiety.

One of the most challenging sides of helping children with anxiety is that anxiety frequently manifests as a collection of undesirable behaviors. Parents and educators are quick to see a problem with behavior, but they do not often notice the underlying anxiety causing it.

This is why I want to share bits of the anxiety world with you. It will help you understand your child's feelings better and connect with them deeper.

Alex's Story

"Knowing what lies ahead, I reluctantly approach the steps of my school.

I feel very lonely, as I do not have any friends here. I always arrive early because I am frightened of being late for class. I could not bear the thought of being late and being scrutinized by everyone.

Because I arrive early, the teachers frequently pass me by. I look down so that we do not have to say "hello" to each other, which would be awkward.

I understand what they are thinking.

'What is the matter with her?'

'Why is it that she has no one to talk to?'

I walk into my first-period class and listen to the conversations around me. Everyone is gushing about how wonderful their weekend was. I keep my head down and try not to draw anyone's attention to myself.

I do the same thing with the teacher, hoping he would not ask me any question. It works some of the time, and sometimes, it does not. When asked a question, I quickly mutter a response, praying the floor would just open up and take me whole.

I frequently have lunch alone or with a group of kids, I used to know but no longer have much in common with. I am sure they are wondering why I am sitting with them since I never say anything. One of them will occasionally ask me a question. I normally keep my gaze fixed on my food and act as if I am not aware of their presence.

Everyone is probably wondering what is wrong with me.

When I have a presentation or a speech, I prepare months ahead of time.

I cannot concentrate for the entire day if it is in my last-period class. My heart is beating so loudly that I am sure everyone can hear it when I finally go up to speak. My hands and voice both tremble. I have a hard time catching my breath. I am sure everyone thinks I am insane or that something is seriously wrong with me.

I have not told anyone how I am feeling because I am too embarrassed and afraid they will think I am making a big deal out of nothing.

Is not it true that I should be able to do these things? It is merely one of my personality flaws that I have problems in social situations. If I work hard enough, I should be able to become more outgoing and capable.

It is kind of odd that I can't talk to anyone about my fear of people since I am terrified of people myself!

Hopefully, I will be able to start over somewhere…, where no one knows me and work through my worries. Perhaps one day, I will get the confidence to seek the help that I need. "

Luna's Story

"My daughter is 11 years old. She has always been a quiet child. Her grades have started to decline this year, even though she has generally done well in school. She has also grown withdrawn and irritable. It hurts me to see her like this.

She will only sit with her two best friends at school, whom she has known since kindergarten. She says that she is terrified of doing anything embarrassing if she hangs around with other girls over lunch or between classes. It began when one of the popular girls mocked Luna about wearing the "wrong" jeans.

She refuses to attend gym class because she does not want to change in front of the other girls and is terrified of making a mistake in class. She has skipped two birthday sleepovers due to a stomachache and refuses to participate in any after-school activities or groups.

Luna's best friends are becoming irritated since she refuses to do anything with them outside of school. When she is with other kids or adults she does not know, I have noticed that she struggles to make eye contact and starts to mumble. This has been going on for about a year, but it has worsened in the last six months. It is breaking my heart, and I do not know what to do."

Henry's Story

"I had already undergone five years of suffering alone with Generalized Anxiety Disorder by the time I was 14 years old.

As I entered my teenage years, the growing weight of anxiety pressing painfully on my chest suffocated my ability to speak up like a smoldering spark. Like a python capturing its victim, the grasp tightened with each attempt I made to break away.

I needed to be free of this enslaving grip. My invisible perpetrator's problem was that I understood very little about its flaws, and I was persuaded that no one else did either.

It is tough to see any way out of this cage when you are lonely and living within the confines of your own head. A black cloud hovers squarely in front of your eyes, casting a pall over any ray of hope.

I began to isolate myself from people who were closest to me. I was afraid of causing harm to others by actions that were beyond my control. I decided to push as many people as possible away from me. It was torturous for me since I could not explain why I was acting in this manner to those who deserved to know the most."

Now that you have an idea of what anxiety feels like and what it can do to your child, it is time to help your child understand it. That is right! He may not even know what he is feeling or why he is feeling it. He needs you to help him.

The most important step is to eliminate anxiety's biggest advantage: its invisibility.

1.2 Helping Your Child Understand Anxiety

Children usually cannot recognize anxiety for what it is. They may instead believe that there is something "wrong" with them. They may become even more worried and self-conscious as a result of these ideas. Teaching your youngster about anxiety and how to spot it is crucial. Self-awareness is important! Here is how you can talk to them about anxiety:

- **Discuss some of your childhood anxieties and how you felt.**

  It is crucial in normalizing conversations about worry and fear. When discussing anxiety with your kids, it is essential to utilize language and scenarios that they can understand.

  If you talk about how you dealt with worry as a youngster and how you applied certain strategies to help you leave the unhelpful thought patterns you had, your kid will feel empowered to deal with their own anxieties.

  Choose your time. Make sure you discuss the physiological indicators of anxiety with your child when he or she is willing to listen.

  Children who discover that they are not alone before they suffer more are more likely to ask for help because they realize it is something they can talk about. They think, "If my parents can talk about how they feel, so can I!"

  When you talk about the time you were terrified or worried, it is better not to anticipate a certain response from your kid in this situation. You are simply trying to establish a link between anxiety and strength.

  If you see that your kid is in pain or if you have a feeling that something is not quite right, you can say,

"Do you recall when I shared about the odd feeling in my stomach and the dizziness I was having?" Have you experienced these feelings?

- **Assist your child in distinguishing between feelings and thoughts.**

  It is critical that you assist younger children in distinguishing between feelings and thoughts so that you can figure out why they are feeling the way they are.

  Your child may believe that "I am scared" is his thought, but this is actually a feeling. You can assist your youngster in identifying the thought that is causing the feeling.

  For example, "The neighbor's dog running around me suggests he might hurt me" could be a logical thought driving the fearful experience.

  Take a seat with your youngster in a comfortable area and talk about taking a moment. Assist them in seeing their thoughts as nothing more than words passing through their heads. They are not the reality, and it is natural for your mind to consider a variety of topics that may happen or not.

- **Explain why we get worried.**

  The sympathetic nervous system or SNS is our internal alarm system, which is also known as the fight-or-flight response.

In real-world alarm circumstances (such as a bear charging at you), the SNS aids communication between your body and brain and, allowing you to respond to the threat by fleeing to safety - or fighting for your life.

Your body's alarm system is attempting to protect you from the threat by activating. When you are in a "fight or flight" state, your body tries to make it simpler for you to run by tightening muscles, raising your heart rate, and changing your breathing pattern.

These modifications allow for higher oxygen levels in the body, which fuels the organs and muscles and helps you survive.

These are some points that will ease your child out of confusion and the worry that tags along.

Chapter 2: Plunging into Anxiety

Let's face it: learning to navigate this massive world while also being the tiniest person in the room most of the time can be terrifying. It can be like being hunted by dinosaurs and monsters beneath the bed.

Not to mention that we rely on "adults" for everything as children, including water, food, and shelter. Let's discuss the possible causes of anxiety in kids in detail.

2.1 But Why?

Anxiety disorders can have complicated causes. Many causes might happen at once, some can lead to others, and some may not always lead to anxiety disorders. However, trauma, school troubles, and/or bullying are examples of environmental stressors leading to mental health issues. Let's go over the major causes one by one:

- **Faster Child Development**

  Many parents and teachers believe that kindergarten is the new first grade. Kindergarten used to be all about finger painting and building blocks thirty years ago. According to a new study, America's kindergarteners have an average of 25 minutes of homework per day. Moreover, first and second graders have three times the amount suggested by the National Education Association. According to a report, in America, time spent in kindergarten on early literacy has increased by 25% since 1998, while time spent on art, physical education, and music has decreased significantly. The higher the grade gets, higher the amount of burden on kids.

- **Overstuffed Schedules**

Overscheduling them for multiple activities or rushing them from place to place might cause stress because children live in the present and like taking the time to experience the world around them. Anxiety is very probable if a parent's schedule or hectic to-do list ignores a child's rhythm.

- **Media Saturation and Adult Content**

Kids are exposed to terrible news stories much younger, thanks to the 24-hour news cycle and constant connectivity. Thanks to smartphones and tablets, today's youth are exposed to more than their fair share of violence and mature sexuality disguised as entertainment, frequently without their parents' knowledge. The use of technological devices is also on the rise.

- **Familial Changes**

Children of all ages might be stressed by major family events such as death, divorce, a parent's job loss, or moving to a new house. The divorce rate in America has been relatively steady over the last decade or so, with approximately 1.5 million children affected by divorce each year. Even the most easygoing youngster might become tense due to heightened emotions, disturbed schedules, and unfamiliar routines. Even pleasant changes, such as the birth of a sibling, can cause anxiety. Stress lingers when there is a considerable change in one's typical routine.

- **Teasing & Bullying**

If you were not invited to a birthday celebration before the Internet, you knew about it, but you didn't have to see photos of the pleasure you missed on Facebook and Instagram. Today's bullying texts are yesterday's cruel letters carried from hand to hand, which have gone global with a single click. Bullying victims, according to research, have more severe anxiety symptoms than others. Bullying has also been connected to social anxiety, which can endure well into adulthood and raise the chance of developing personality disorders.

- **Fewer Outlets for Stress**

Do you remember recess? Your children may disagree. According to a report, 8% of third-graders and 7% of first-graders do not have recess in America. Since 2008, 20 percent of American school districts have reduced recess time by 50 minutes per week on average. Physical education has been reduced as well. PE is usually only done once or twice a week for most children.

- **Losing Sleep**

School stresses and the allure of social media eat away at an essential stress reliever: sleep. According to the National Sleep Foundation, one-third of parents believe schoolwork and after-school activities interfere with their children's sleep. Nearly three out of every four children aged six to seventeen have at least one electronic device in their bedroom, which can shorten a night's sleep by nearly an hour. Even minor sleep loss has been shown to influence memory, judgment, and mood in studies.

- **Parental Stress**

  A child's stress buffer is his or her family. However, when a family is struggling and unable to fulfill this function, a youngster is under even greater stress. As parents, we know how easily we can get into a rut when all we can think about are 'the next 20 things I need to do.' You can relieve tension and regain energy for the next assignment by just spending some unstructured time with your children.

- **Puberty**

  Experiencing physical changes and/or reaching puberty can be distressing. This period is full of unsettling unknowns and, in some situations, awkwardness, both of which can cause stress.

These are some causes of anxiety for kids under 12. Let's discuss a huge factor in a child's anxiety separately. It will include the various ways parents can unknowingly cause or spiral their kid's anxiety out of control.

2.2 Parental Habits and Anxiety Oxygen

As parents, we can either be a part of the problem or a part of the solution. And we are in the wrong camp more often than we would like to acknowledge.

Although it is not your fault if your child is anxious, some of the parenting techniques you are proudest of or your personal habits may actually be flaming up the problem.

- **Anxious Talk**

    At all the wrong times, children are master listeners. While you may find yourself repeating the same instructions to no avail, you may also discover that the time your children tune in, coincides with the time you believe you are having a private chat with another adult.

    It is vital to talk about your worries with someone who will listen and help you work them out. Still, it is also important to remember that children have a tendency to fill in the gaps on their own when they hear small bits of potentially frightening information. Talking to your friends about your fears of a school shooting is healthy, but discussing this subject with your children before or near them can exacerbate their anxieties and concerns.

    By observing them, children might internalize their parents' anxieties, worries, and anxious talk.

- **Over Shielding**

  Negative parenting actions that cause anxiety, can include attempts to protect children from all potential danger. Shielding children during play can include frequent reminders to be careful while playing and imposing limits on how high they can climb or where they can leap from. The message is clear: playing is risky, and you will get hurt.

  Kids must take healthy risks to realize what they are capable of and learn how to make good decisions. When parents protect their children from prospective threats that may or may not exist, children develop a fear of taking risks.

- **Caring a Bit Too Much**

  You feel bad for your child when she comes home from school with stories about mean fellows and insensitive teachers, and you often express it, but you should not. Kids feed off of our emotions and become more distressed when we are. When my daughter expresses her concerns to me, only for me to get concerned as well, it exacerbates the situation. She expects me to be strong, but instead, I transmit the message that anxiousness is the 'correct' response to her challenges. We must keep our own concerns in check while sympathizing with theirs, no matter how difficult it is. We must be the emotional rock: the person who understands, supports, and, if requested, advises others without ever revealing that our own difficulties cause us anxiety.

- **Avoidance Behavior**

  If certain fears make you uncomfortable, you may respond by avoiding them. You may even back this up by repeatedly mentioning the source of the anxiety. If you cross the street any time you see a dog, you may mention being bitten by a dog when you were a tiny child to explain why you think dogs are unpredictable. This is a common response to a fear that is based on prior experience. The problem is that children pick up on their parents' avoidance practices. In this scenario, the message they hear is that all dogs are frightening and unpredictable and should be avoided.

  It takes time and practice to work through specific phobias. To prevent sharing your concerns with your children, enlist the support of your spouse or another adult in their lives to ensure that your children are exposed to your triggers in a healthy way that does not set off the alarm system. If your children are afraid of dogs, your spouse could take them to a pet adoption event where they can see and pet dogs and cats to help them become accustomed to the fear of the unknown.

- **Compensating Behavior**

  We all want to assist our children with their weaknesses. We hire a tutor after one bad math grade. We get them a book about coping with bullies after an incident. However, we are unintentionally teaching kids to focus on the negative. Most of us gain confidence by playing to our strengths rather than adjusting for our flaws. Those who are truly content with our adult life have learned to focus on what we are good at while ignoring the rest. The things we are really poor at are probably delegated or outsourced. Although children cannot always avoid their weak areas, concentrating on their strengths helps them to develop self-efficacy and confidence. If you are tempted to spend the weekend looking for math tutors because your child is struggling with arithmetic, spend the weekend doing things he enjoys. His self-assurance and skill will resurface. It may carry over to his next math lesson.

- **Harsh Parenting**

In an age where the recipe for success appears to be eternally regressive — when a successful career involves acing your way through a good high school, middle school, and even preschool — the obligation is to push, push, push. We want these little humans to be able to get their foot in the door before they even learn how to tie shoes on their own. According to new research, parents who chastise their children harshly may be saddling them with anxiety that lasts a lifetime. Researchers collected childhood memories from over 4,000 persons of various ages and connected them with the participants' self-reported mental health in a survey released last November. According to the findings, children raised by authoritarian parents have a tougher time adapting to misfortune later in life.

- **Over Advocating**

  We all want to advocate for our children, yet our willingness to do so can sometimes increase worry. When your kid confides in you about a school issue, your first instinct is to march into the school and try to solve it. This conveys two messages to your youngster. For starters, he cannot tell you things in confidence, and you do not trust him to solve his own difficulties. Make it clear to the little ones that you will only campaign on their behalf with their permission and knowledge. Your first aim should always be to help them in finding a solution that they can implement without your assistance.

Anxiety may have a negative impact on everything from school to physical health and relationships. Learning to recognize your triggers and develop effective coping strategies helps you control your anxious thinking cycle and teaches your children that they can find a way to deal with their own triggers and fight through the ups and downs that come with growing up.

2.3 Anxiety Evaluation in my Child

Parents frequently state that they knew their child was different from a young age but did not recognize it as an anxiety problem. Some parents hoped that their child would "grow out of it," never anticipating that their youngster would become even more impairing over time. Other parents saw the worried behaviors as normal since they acted anxiously.

Parents of children with anxiety are often perplexed, frustrated, and overwhelmed. The guide below is to help you figure out if your child has anxiety and clear this confusion.

Anxiety has many complex symptoms that vary greatly from child to child. Following are some symptoms that your child may be suffering from an anxiety disorder:

- Sleeping problems

- Keeping away from certain circumstances

- Mood swings, stomachaches, and other bodily aches and pains

- Being clinging in the presence of parents or caregivers

- Tantrums

- Having difficulty concentrating in class or being extremely fidgety

- Being extremely self-aware

Depending on what they are most concerned about, children can be diagnosed with various types of anxiety. Look out for the signs mentioned with these anxiety disorders.

Generalized Anxiety Disorder

Children with generalized anxiety disorder are concerned about a wide range of issues. Their anxiety is unrelated to anything specific, yet it is severe enough to interfere with daily life.

Signs and symptoms of generalized anxiety disorder in children are:

- Feeling tense

- Restlessness

- Fatigued all the time

- Feeling enraged

- Concentration issues

- Sleeping problems

Children must have symptoms on most days for at least six months to be diagnosed with generalized anxiety disorder.

Social Anxiety Disorder

Youngsters with social anxiety disorder are excessively self-conscious when it comes to other people. They avoid social situations and even speak in class because they are afraid of embarrassment.

The signs of social anxiety disorder in children are:

- Avoiding most social settings, feeling bad when they have to participate in them.

- In social circumstances, physical symptoms such as shivering, sweating, or difficulty breathing

- Tantrums and sobbing in social circumstances

- Fear of others condemning them because of their anxiety

A child's fear would be so severe that it interferes with daily life for them to be diagnosed with social anxiety disorder.

Separation Anxiety Disorder

When youngsters are separated from their parents or caregivers, they become tremendously distressed. This anxiousness is a lot more than what other kids of their age experience.

Separation anxiety manifests itself in the ways like:

- Concerned about parents or caregivers getting ill or dying.

- Refusing to go to school or leave the house

- Fear of falling asleep or being alone

- Separation-related nightmares

- Physical signs of impending separation (such as headaches or stomachaches)

Separation anxiety disorder affects children for at least four weeks.

Selective Mutism

Selective Mutism makes it difficult for children to talk in some contexts, such as at school. These are not just shy children; their anxiousness is so severe that they are paralyzed and unable to talk.

To get a selective mutism diagnosis, the kid must:

- Be able to speak in some situations but not in others.

- Have this issue for at least a month.

- Having trouble with school and social activities.

If a communication impairment or a language barrier is the source of a child's difficulty speaking, it is not labeled as selective mutism.

Obsessive-Compulsive Disorder

Children with OCD have anxiety-inducing ideas and worries. They create rules for themselves that they believe they must adhere to manage their anxiety.

- Compulsions are the rules that children believe they must follow to overcome their anxieties.

- Obsessions are unwanted thoughts that cause distress and anxiety in children.

When a child has obsessions, compulsions, or both, they may be diagnosed with OCD.

Panic Attacks

Panic attacks occur frequently and unexpectedly in children with panic disorder. Physical symptoms of panic episodes might lead children to believe they are dying or suffering a heart attack. When a child has at least one panic episode and exhibits other symptoms, they are diagnosed with panic disorder.

- Fear of having more panic attacks

- After the panic episodes, they change their behavior dramatically, such as avoiding places that remind them of the event.

When a specialist diagnoses a child with panic disorder, they rule out medical factors and other issues such as PTSD.

Specific Phobia

Specific phobias affect children who are terrified of one or more specific objects. This is a fear of something that is not usually dangerous. Phobias cause problems in children's lives because they go to great lengths to avoid what they are scared of.

The following are examples of common childhood phobias:

- Insects or animals

- Natural elements like heights and water

- Blood

- Specific situations like crowds or confined areas

- Other symptoms include choking, vomiting, or hearing loud noises.

I want to add even if your child does not classify for an anxiety disorder, it still means that he needs your attention as he could be leaning towards a particular disorder.

Chapter 3: Crippling with Anxiety

A healthy dose of anxiety can act as motivation. It can assist one in focusing on a goal to complete a task or attain achievement. For example, if your young one is nervous about a test, he may study more to pass the exam. An appropriate level of anxiety promotes growth, development, and the acquisition of new abilities. However, an unhealthy amount of anxiety can have terrible effects on kids. Let's discuss the major possibilities.

3.1 Poor Learning and School Performance

Anxiety can affect a child's capacity to learn in various ways.

Anxiety has been found to have a noticeable impact on our working memory in studies. When people are worried, they have a harder time remembering things. Anxiety's unpleasantness and pervasive presence tend to trump other cognitive functions.

Anxiety impacts a child's entire mental process, not just his memory. Anxiety, as previously stated, tends to take precedence over other cognitive processes. This implies that when your child is stressed, they may be unable to think clearly. When socializing with other students, this can make it difficult for them to follow a lesson, give answers to queries, or compose phrases. All of these difficulties can have a negative impact on your child's academic performance.

Children are irritated by anxiety. It is especially true given how difficult it is for a toddler to recognize anxiety. If you have ever struggled with anxiety, you are probably aware of how long it took you to recognize it for what it was.

Unfortunately, most children do not yet have a name for their unusual feelings of unease and dissatisfaction. It makes it harder for them to communicate and may cause them to become irritated.

Naturally, children do not like to be anxious. They are inclined to make great efforts to avoid circumstances that cause them anxiety. If they are worried at school, they may be more likely to skip classes. They may also avoid doing homework or make-up excuses to avoid doing it.

Parents frequently ignore children's concerns because they lack the ability to easily explain why they do not want to go to school. After all, it makes them anxious. Despite their nervousness, children forced to attend school may develop resentments, and their anxiety may worsen.

Closely review your child's report cards and progress reports. Low grades could also indicate an anxiety issue. This is particularly true if your child's grades have declined.

An anxious adolescent may frequently postpone and miss assignments. They may eventually begin skipping classes or refuse to attend school at all. Anxious students have a hard time focusing their attention. As a result, they may be unable to meet their academic objectives.

However, keep in mind that many worried teenagers perform well in school. Their academic performance is often comparable to that of non-anxious youngsters. They do, however, take longer to complete jobs.

3.2 Social Withdrawal

Anxious children, particularly those with social anxiety disorder, may isolate themselves. They do it to avoid social interaction's stress. A psychiatrist, Dr. Ashley Miller, explained that social interaction is even more important for kids and teens than adults because it influences their brain development.

Social isolation, in turn, causes more anxiety. Isolation causes a person to become more internalized. As a result, their minds get distracted by negative thoughts. Anxiety can make it challenging for a person to see the world through other people's eyes. So, it may be tougher for anxiety sufferers to build new empathetic relationships.

Examine your child's social behaviors to evaluate if they have altered considerably. Here are a few examples of specific conduct to watch out for:

- Not participating in extracurricular activities

- Friendship interactions are fewer.

- Having to spend more time alone than usual

3.3 Sleep Disturbances

A child of 7-12 years old should have 10 hours of sleep every night.

There are various reasons why a little one may not be getting enough sleep. It includes exposure to electronics because blue light affects melatonin secretion. In other instances, the condition could be linked to anxiety. Anxiety can not only cause sleep deprivation, but it also is the other way around. As a result, it very well has the potential to spiral out of control.

Sleep disturbances are one of the most common anxiety symptoms. This problem can manifest itself in a lot of ways, including the inability to fall asleep, waking up repeatedly due to worrying thoughts, exhaustion when awake, and unsatisfying sleep. Anxiety makes you think about the same bad thoughts repeatedly with no end in sight. You are most likely to continue thinking about all of your worries while you fall asleep. Because of your anxiety, you worry about the tiniest things and exaggerate them, resulting in insomnia.

As a result of your anxiousness, you may have frightening nightmares. Rapid eye movement (REM) sleep, which allows you to have vivid dreams, can be provoked by anxiety. It might cause you to experience more vivid and unsettling dreams, disrupting your sleep even more. You may develop a phobia of falling asleep, upsetting your sleep schedule and routine.

Sleep anxiety is a condition that some people experience due to their inability to fall asleep. Due to your difficulties falling and keeping asleep, you may dread going to bed at night since you know you'll be tormented by your nervous thoughts for the rest of the night. This form of anticipatory worry can further disrupt your sleep schedule.

Keep a close check on your child's sleeping habits. Keep an eye out for the following red flags:

- Staying up late at night

- Having a hard time getting out of bed in the morning

- Feeling drowsy during the day

Put away all electronic devices in the room at least half an hour before night. Keep an eye on your child's behavior to see whether it improves.

3.4 Low Self-Esteem

Self-esteem is defined as our overall view or evaluation of ourselves, including our judgments about ourselves and the value we attach to ourselves. Most children's self-esteem will have ups and downs as they progress through life's phases and obstacles. They will be subjected to various pressures, including social media, bullying, exams, family problems, and abuse.

However, children with a general anxiety disorder or social anxiety may struggle much more with low self-esteem. They can develop other issues, such as adolescent depression. If your child has low self-esteem, he may constantly doubt their abilities or knowledge. He might also go to considerable efforts to win others' approval. Here are some more signs of poor self-esteem:

- Tend to avoid new and unusual situations.

- Tend to put themselves down, saying things like "I'm stupid" or "I won't be able to achieve that" (before even trying).
- Are unable to cope effectively with failure in general.
- Have the impression that their efforts are never nearly as good as others'.
- Have a negative tendency to compare themselves to their age fellows.

Keep an eye on your adolescent's self-perception. If he puts himself down or reacts adversely to criticism, he has low self-esteem. He could have an anxiety problem.

3.5 Panic Attacks

A panic attack is a sign of panic disorder, a type of anxiety disorder. Contrary to popular misconception, this condition is not like an anxiety attack. Anxiety attacks usually come on gradually as a result of stressful situations. Panic episodes, on the other hand, strike without warning and are typically accompanied by a sense of impending death. However, many of the symptoms of panic attacks and anxiety attacks are the same. Some of the most common ones to be aware of are:

- Sweating
- Discomfort or pain in the chest
- Dry mouth
- Faster heart rate
- Tightness in the throat
- Breathing problems
- Fear
- Tingling or numbness

- Nausea
- Dizziness

If you notice indicators of a panic or anxiety attack in your child, take him to a professional.

3.6 Unhealthy Eating Habits

According to psychologist Susan Albers, there is a link between anxiety and appetite, but it is not the same for everyone. Some people are prone to ignoring their hunger cues and refraining from eating for long periods due to stress. Others become emotional eaters who eat mindlessly as a result of stress.

When you are worried, your body produces cortisol, also known as the stress hormone. Because your brain believes it requires fuel to fight whatever threat is generating the stress, cortisol can make you crave sweet, salty, and greasy meals.

It has also been shown in studies to impact your metabolism. According to a recent study, participants who communicated one or more stressors in the previous 24 hours, such as disagreements with friends, trouble with children, arguments with spouses, or work-related pressures, burned 104 lesser calories in the 7 hours after eating a high in fat meal than non-stressed participants.

Moreover, anxiety in children is usually associated with stomach trouble. This might result in a loss of appetite and a reduction in the amount of food consumed by a youngster. Low food intake can become problematic if it leads to low body weight or failure to attain the weight a child need for optimal growth and development.

Lastly, according to studies, children who are very picky about what they eat are more prone to worry and anxiety. So unhealthy eating habits and anxiety form a painful and hard to escape cycle.

3.7 Impaired Bodily Function

Digestive Function

Anxiety has an impact on human digestive and excretory systems. Stomachaches, nausea, diarrhea, and other digestive problems occur as a result. It can even make you lose your appetite causing weight loss with other complications that tag along with it.

Anxiety disorders have been linked to irritable bowel syndrome (IBS) development following a bowel infection. Vomiting, diarrhea, and constipation are all symptoms of IBS.

Immunity Function

Anxiety can activate your fight-or-flight stress response, which releases chemicals and hormones into your system, including adrenaline. If you are nervous and stressed regularly or for an extended period, your body will not receive the signal to get back to normal functioning. It can cause your immune system to deteriorate, making you more susceptible to viral infections and diseases. Additionally, your usual immunizations may not perform as well if you have anxiety.

Respiratory Function

Hyperventilation occurs when a person's breathing becomes quick and shallow during times of anxiety. Hyperventilation permits the lungs to take in more oxygen and distribute it more swiftly throughout the body. Extra oxygen aids the body's preparation for combat or flight.

People who are hyperventilating may feel as though they are not getting enough oxygen and may gasp for air. This can exacerbate hyperventilation and its associated symptoms, such as:

- Feeling faint
- Dizziness
- Lightheadedness
- Weakness
- Tingling

Moreover, anxiety can negatively affect the cardiovascular system increasing the risk of heart diseases.

3.8 Impaired Brain Function

Bigger Amygdala

Anxiety can cause your brain to become hypersensitive to threats. Your amygdala expands when you suffer from anxiety regularly. The amygdala is a little almond-shaped structure in the limbic system, which is the region of your brain that controls moods and emotions. The amygdala acts as a watchdog in your brain, always scanning for danger. When the amygdala detects a threat, it sends a signal to the hypothalamus, triggering the fight or flight response. The amygdala is a big and hypersensitive structure in the anxious brain. As a result, the amygdala generates a lot of wrong alarms. An over active amygdala can be compared to a watchman who barks too much. The hyperactive amygdala sends out so many false alarms that your brain perceives risks even in non-risky situations. That is why persons with anxiety issues are more likely to feel threatened than those who do not.

Shrunk Hippocampus

Your body is stressed out when you have anxiety. The hippocampus, the portion of the brain that stores long-term and contextual memory, shrinks due to stress. It may become more challenging for your brain to hold onto memories as the hippocampus shrinks. But here is the catch: anxiety fools the hippocampus into believing that anxiety-related memories are safe to keep and recall. As a result, the few memories you do retain will be those associated with anxiety. In other words, anxiety reprograms your brain to recall failure, threat, and danger. Memories of achievement, success, and safety, for example, are buried deep in the basement of your brain.

Weakened Bridges

The connections between the PFC (Prefrontal Cortex) and the amygdala are weakened by anxiety. The PFC should kick in and assist you in coming up with a logical and rational reaction when the amygdala warns the brain of danger. The PFC guarantees that you can analyze data analytically, make well-informed decisions, and assist you in problem-solving. The PFC might be thought of as your brain's wise counselor. In brains free of anxiety, when the amygdala sounds alarms, the prefrontal cortex replies rationally. Anxious brains are not the same. The connection between the PFC and amygdala is weak when the amygdala warns the PFC of danger. As a result, the problem-solving rational section of the brain is silenced, leading to irrational thinking and chaotic behavior.

Lastly, your baseline level of anxiety may rise if excessive amounts of stress hormones flood the brain repeatedly. You could progress from mild anxiety, which most of us deal with on a daily basis, to moderate anxiety. Moderate anxiety is a little more acute and overwhelming, and it makes you uneasy and agitated all of the time. If your brain continues to be extremely sensitive to anxiety, your anxiety level may rise to the point where you cannot think properly.

These are major ways your child can fight his battle with anxiety. Let's enter into our practical section of the book to deal with this problem head-on.

Chapter 4: Worry Toolkit

According to Penn State University experts, just approximately 8% of the things people worry about come true. In other words, just roughly one out of every ten things you worry about is actually worth it.

Worry might feel productive at times. It can feel lazy to take time to relax and stop worrying about what's bothering you - and it can even make you worry more! Even if it appears that staying stressed is the easier option, you will be happier in the long term if you make an effort to learn how to stop worrying.

So how can you help your child worry less? Below are some parental strategies to help your child with excessive worrying.

4.1 Connect with Sympathy

Encourage them to speak their minds. Make an effort to communicate with your child. Inquire about their day and the things they did. It could be as easy as inviting them to help you with a task, such as cooking dinner, so you can catch up on each other's lives.

Remind them that you are always available for them and that you are interested in their thoughts and feelings. A few encouraging words can help them feel more at ease about sharing their emotions with you.

It is critical to notice and comprehend the sentiments that your child is experiencing, even if it is uncomfortable for you. When they share their feelings with you, you can reply with "I understand. It seems like a bad situation," or "that makes sense.

It is easy to notice things your child does that you do not like. Try to acknowledge and commend them on something they are doing well, even if it is something as little as picking up after themselves.

Take the time to express your love for them. Work together to build new routines and attainable daily goals. You might plan your domestic tasks around your academics or establish a goal, such as finishing your homework before dinner.

Allow enough time and space for your child to be independent. It is a normal part of growing up to need more space.

Find a few ideas to help and encourage your kid to take time away from schoolwork, housework, or other tasks to do something they enjoy. Work with your little one to come up with some problem-solving suggestions if they are frustrated. Make a conscious effort to avoid taking authority and telling them what to do.

To settle disagreements, work together. Listen to your child's viewpoints and try to resolve disagreements in a calm manner. Keep in mind that stress affects everyone.

When you are angry, you should not talk about it. Take a step back, inhale deeply, and relax; you can talk to your teen about it later. Regardless of the circumstances, power battles should be avoided. Empathize with their desire to maintain control in a stressful circumstance, no matter how difficult it may be at the time, rather than fighting back or being overwhelmed.

Be open and honest with them. You can even tell your child if you are stressed out. Demonstrating how you deal with difficult emotions might persuade children that theirs are normal. Take some moments to think about how you and your child will deal with a problem if one develops. You can tell your child about your thoughts and point of view about a subject so they can mature their mindset.

4.2 Create a Worry Dump Period

Little ones, when anxiety and concern take over your thoughts and distract you from school, or your personal life, it is difficult to be effective in your everyday tasks. This is when the worry-deferral approach comes in handy. Allow yourself to experience an anxious thought rather than trying to stop or get rid of it. Instead of obsessing about it, permit yourself to have it.

- Make a "worry period" for your kids. Set up a specific time and location with their help for worrying. It should be the same every day, e.g., from 6:00 to 6:20 p.m. in the living room) and start early enough that it would not make your kid nervous right before night. Your kid is free to worry about anything that is on their mind during their worry period. The remainder of the day, on the other hand, is worry-free.

- Help your child make a list of their concerns. If an anxious thought or worry enters their mind during the day, ask them to write it down quickly and move on with their day. Remind them that they will have time to think about it later, so do not stress about it now. Furthermore, writing down their thoughts — whether on a pad or their computer — is far more difficult than merely thinking them, so their anxieties are more likely to fade away.

- During the worry period, help them go over their "worry list." Allow your kids to worry about the thoughts they wrote down if the worries continue to trouble them, but only for the length of time, they have set aside for their worry period. They will typically find it easier to build a more balanced viewpoint as they explore their issues in this way. If their worries do not seem essential any longer, simply ask them to go about their day.

4.2 Validate Feelings

It is easy to say things like, "Oh, it is not a big deal," "Don't worry about it," or "You're going to be OK," when your child expresses concern about something. Such reactions provide the message that your child's sentiments are wrong.

Instead, confirm their feelings by saying something like, "It seems like you are nervous right now," or "I would be nervous too if I had to speak in front of a large crowd."

Then, despite their nerves, write a message expressing your confidence in their ability to achieve. "It is difficult to undertake scary things like this," say, "but I am convinced you can do it."

Make sure you are saying something along the lines of, "It's alright to be terrified, and you can choose to be brave and strong," rather than, "You shouldn't be nervous."

The most crucial validation guideline is to avoid using the word "but." Your youngster will feel unheard if you say, "I hear you're worried, but you'll be fine." Instead of trying to fix your child's grief, ignore your natural reaction and simply validate their feelings. Use the word "and" when delivering soothing ideas, so your child understands they have been heard, AND you can provide them with correct information to feel more in control of the issue. For example:

"I can tell you're concerned about Grandma. I'm in the same boat. I phone her to say hello and tell her that I miss her when I'm worried about her. For now, we will not meet Grandma to help her stay well, as we have been instructed to. We're doing everything we can to keep Grandma well. So, the only thing left is to reach out to her as much as possible to ensure she doesn't feel alone. She likes it when we talk with her; it makes her very happy. Is there anything you'd like to do to let Grandma know you're thinking about her?"

Lastly, respect their emotions, but do not give them power. It is critical to realize that validation does not always imply agreement. So, if a youngster is scared of going to the doctor for a shot, you do not want to dismiss their anxieties, but you also do not want to exaggerate them. You should listen and be empathic, as well as help them comprehend what they are worried about and urge them to face their worries. You should say, "I know you're terrified, and that's okay. I'm here, and I'm going to help you get through this."

4.4 Distinguish between Real vs. False Alarms

Discuss with your youngster how anxiety serves to keep them safe. For example, if a lion was hunting them, their brain would send a warning signal to their body. They might experience physical changes such as sweaty palms and a faster heart rate. As they were ready to flee from the lion, they would feel a surge of energy (a real threat).

Then inform them that their brain can also set up a false warning at times. They may experience great panic as a result of these false alarms, even if the scenario isn't life-or-death. Examples of false alarms are situations such as trying out for the basketball team, speaking in front of a large group, or preparing for a huge test.

"Is your brain sending you a real alert right now or a false alarm?" question them when they are anxious. Then, assist them in deciding what course of action to take.

Explain that if there is a serious threat, they should pay attention to the warning signs and take steps to protect themselves. If it is a false alarm, though, it is a good idea to confront their worries.

4.5 Change Thought Pattern

Your child, like adults, is prone to negative thinking. This kind of negative thinking can make them feel anxious and lower their self-esteem.

You may educate them on how to identify negative thoughts, question them, and use positive self-talk to convert them into positive, realistic ones.

- **Recognize It**

  Your kids must first be able to recognize a negative thought before they may address it. Assist them in making a shortlist of unpleasant thoughts that they frequently have.

- **Challenge It**

  Encourage your youngster to think of themselves as a detective, gathering evidence to evaluate the evidence behind their worrisome thoughts. For instance, if they often tell themselves, "I am stupid," they should ask themselves, "Is it true that I'm stupid? Have there been times when I showed my intelligence?" This will teach them not to believe every bad thought that enters their mind.

- **Change It**

  The final phase is to replace their negative self-talk with a positive one after recognizing and challenging it. "Oh honey, you're not stupid," do not say right away. They will not only refuse to trust you, but they will also refuse to learn how to change their negative thinking. Instead, say, "What would you say to a friend who thought he was stupid?" Encourage them to tell themselves the same thing when they respond with kindness.

You can teach your children new thinking methods to help them turn their worries into reassurances. Replace "I'm worried that my mom won't pick me up from school" with "I know my mom will pick me up from school since she ALWAYS does." You can say each worry out loud together and come up with fresh statements to counter the old. Practice these with your children until they become routine substitutes for the old, nagging fears. This is a crucial ability in the development of resilience.

Lastly, while reassuring an anxious youngster is crucial, it is even more important to educate them on how to treat themselves with care and compassion by adopting healthier self-talk. They can then reassure themselves while you are not by their side to offer encouraging remarks.

4.6 Distinguish between Solvable vs. Non-solvable Worries

Problem-solving entails assessing a situation, making clear strategies to address it, and putting the plan into action. Worrying, however, almost never results in a solution. You are no more equipped to deal with worst-case scenarios if they actually happen, no matter how many hours you spend thinking about them.

Teach your child the difference between worries that can have a solution and worries that do not have any.

Worries that are productive and solvable can be addressed straight away. If you are concerned about your bills, for example, you could contact your creditors to inquire about more flexible payment choices. Worries that are unproductive and insoluble have no matching action. "What if I develop cancer?" or "What if my child has an accident?"

- Ask your child to start brainstorming if the problem is solvable. Make a list of all the potential solutions that come to mind. Do not get too caught up in finding the ideal solution. Concentrate on the things they can change rather than the events or facts beyond their control. Make a plan of action after they have analyzed their choices. They will feel a lot better once they have made a plan and started working on the problem.

  For instance, your child has a presentation on Monday. Instead of worrying about it, ask your child what can he do to solve the problem? Help him come up with solutions, e.g., working on speech skills, researching the subject and practice, etc.

- Help your child accept the uncertainty if the worry is unsolvable. Worrying is a common technique for them to foretell what the future holds to avoid unpleasant surprises and exert influence over the outcome. The issue is that it does not work. It does not make life any more predictable to think about all the things that could go wrong. Focusing on the worst-case situations can prevent you from appreciating the nice things you have now. Help them answer these questions:

  ➤ Do you tend to predict terrible things just because they are uncertain? What are the chances that they will?

> ➤ Given the low probability, is it okay to live with the slight risk that something bad would happen?

> ➤ How do your parents deal with uncertainty in different scenarios? Would you be able to do the same?

Help your children pay attention to your emotions. Teach them emotional intelligence. Worrying about uncertainty is a common coping mechanism for people who want to avoid unpleasant emotions. However, by becoming more aware of your emotions, you might begin to embrace them, even if they are unpleasant or illogical.

4.7 Personify Your Child's Worry

As you surely know by now, ignoring anxiety does not help but binging fear to life and talking about it like an actual person can. Make a character for your child who is worried. For example, Og (an imaginary character) is the embodiment of fear. Og lives in the part of the brain that keeps us safe while we are in danger. Of course, Og may go out of hand at times, and when that happens, we have to speak some sense into him. A similar idea can be used on a plush animal or even role-playing at home.

There are several advantages to personifying worry or creating a character. It can help children understand the frightening physical response when they are worried. It can stimulate the logical brain, and it is a strategy that your child can practice at any moment.

4.8 Create a Relaxation Kit

When you are stressed, what do you like to do? De-stressing can mean taking a long bubble bath or curling up with a nice book. Others prefer to go for a leisurely jog on a natural route or simply spend time with their dog at the local dog park.

It is often beneficial to be a little more organized with children. You can put together a "relaxation kit" with toys, games, or other items to help your youngster refocus and relax. Fill a box with coloring books, fidget toys, a beloved plush animal, or even kinetic sand or clay for a go-to relaxation kit.

4.9 Go from 'What If' to 'What is'

Humans can travel through time, which you may not be aware of. In truth, we spend a lot of mental energy planning for the future. This form of mental time travel can increase anxiety in people who already have it. What-if scenarios are common among time travelers: "What if I cannot access my locker and miss class?" "What if Suzy refuses to speak with me today?"

According to research, returning to the present can help ease this urge. Mindfulness exercises are one excellent way to accomplish this. A child's mind is brought from "what if" to "what is" through mindfulness. Simply assist your youngster focus on their breath for a few minutes to do this. Here are a few exercises to teach your kid.

Bunnies, flowers, snakes, and candles are among the imagery used in these exercises to stimulate active imaginations. We want youngsters to like these exercises so they should be fun. If your child enjoys hissing like a snake or is charmed by the fragrance of flowers, feel free to choose whichever method inspires them the most. Use as needed and repeat until your youngster is relaxed or settled down enough to talk about their feelings.

- Imagine inhaling the smell of a flower. Inhale through your nose. Exhale through your mouth.

- Take three short sniffs through the nose, and one deep exhale through the nose for the Bunny Breath. (As she gets the hang of it, have your tiny bunny concentrate on slowing down the exhale.)

- Inhale gently through your nose. Exhale slowly through your mouth with a long, slow hissing sound.

- Imagine a birthday candle being blown out. To blow out the candle, take a deep breath in through your nose and then exhale through your mouth.

- Blow out the Candle/Smell the Rose: Combine the smell the rose (SR) on the inhale and with the Blow Out the Candle (BC) on the exhale by putting your pointer finger to your nose to "SR" and dropping your finger to your lips to "BC."

Teaching children the "bubble blowing" method is another option. Tell them to act like they are using a wand to blow bubbles. Remind them that they need to blow softly to obtain a huge bubble. This will help them remember to exhale slowly.

4.10 Motivate Them to Move Their Body

Incorporate exercise in your child's daily routine. If they require assistance, practice with them. Exercise releases endorphins, which lower stress and tension, increase energy, and improve your overall sense of well-being, making it a natural and effective anti-anxiety medication. More importantly, by focusing on how your body feels while walking, you can stop the cycle of anxiety going through your head. Ask them to focus on how their feet are on the ground, the rhythm of their breathing, or the feel of the sun or breeze on their skin while they walk, run, or dance.

Swimming, hiking, soccer, shooting baskets, dodge ball, martial arts, tennis, jumping rope, bicycling, rock climbing, gymnastics, dance, or yoga are examples of activities that your youngster may like. Any activity that raises your child's heart rate will help in the battle against the Worry Monster.

4.11 Work through a Checklist

When faced with an emergency, what do trained pilots do? They do not just go with the flow; they consult their emergency plans. Even after years of training, every pilot goes through a checklist because it is difficult to think properly when you are in danger.

When children experience anxiety, they experience it in the same way as adults. Why not make a checklist to give them a step-by-step plan for calming down? What do you want them to do if they start to feel anxious? If they benefit from breathing, the first step is to pause and breathe. They can then assess the situation. Finally, you may print out a checklist for your child to refer to whenever they are worried.

4.12 Avoid Avoiding Anxiety

Do your kids want to avoid social situations, school, pets, aircraft, or anything else that makes them nervous? Do you, as a parent, help them in doing so? Yes, of course! This is entirely natural. The flight component of the flight-fight-freeze response encourages your children to flee the danger. Unfortunately, avoidance exacerbates worry in the long run.

So, what is the other option? Consider using a technique known as laddering—kids can manage their anxiety by breaking it down into manageable bits. To achieve the goal, laddering employs the chunking principle and incremental exposure.

Let's imagine your kid is terrified of riding the park's swings. Create mini-goals to move closer to the larger goal instead of avoiding it (e.g., go to the park's edge, then walk into the park, go to the swings, and, then, get on a swing). You may use each step until the exposure becomes too simple; at that point, it is time to climb up the ladder to the next rung.

4.13 Provide Distractions

Provide a good distraction for your children. Allow them to choose a favorite activity, such as ten minutes on the internet playing a mental game, a time out for reading a beloved book, watching a half-hour television show, or going for a little bike ride around the block, and undertake that exercise whenever a worry attack strikes. This lets them combat worry with pleasure, diverting their attention away from the Worry Monster's often paralyzing thoughts and feelings. They have been distracted from their troubles before you, even realizing it.

4.14 Stop Reinforcing Worries

Encourage your child to express their emotions, but refrain from asking leading questions like, "Are you nervous about the big test?" "Do you have any concerns about the science fair?" Simply use open-ended inquiries, such as, "How are you feeling about the science fair?" to avoid perpetuating the anxiety loop.

Furthermore, by your tone of voice or body language, you do not want to imply that "Perhaps this is something you should be terrified of." Consider the case of a child who has had a bad experience with a dog. You might be afraid about how they will react the next time they are around a dog, and you might unwittingly transmit the message that they should be concerned.

4.15 Encourage Tolerance

Let your youngster realize how much effort it takes to overcome worry to accomplish what they want or need to do. It is very motivating for them to get involved in life and let the worry flow naturally. It is called the "habituation curve." As he maintains contact with the stressor, it will decrease with time. It may not reach zero or drop as soon as you would like, but that is how we overcome our worries.

4.16 Help Them See Worry Differently

Chronic worrying is the most common symptom of GAD (Generalized Anxiety Disorder). It is critical to comprehend what worrying is because your child's worry beliefs have a significant part in the onset and maintenance of GAD. Your kids may believe that your problems stem from the outside world—from other people, stressful events, or challenging situations. Worry, on the other hand, is self-created. Although the trigger is external, their internal running dialogue keeps it going.

When they worry, they are talking to themselves about the things they are frightened of or potential negative situations. They mentally go over the feared circumstance and consider all possible responses. In other words, they are attempting to fix problems that have not yet occurred, or, even worse, they are merely dwelling on worst-case possibilities.

All of their worrying could make you think they are protecting yourself by preparing for the worst or avoiding unfavorable situations. On the other hand, worrying is typically ineffective, draining their mental and emotional energy without yielding any tangible problem-solving solutions or activities.

4.17 Model Effective Worry Tackling

It is no surprise that one of the key explanations for children's conduct is their parents' behavior. The majority of the times, youngsters imitate the actions of their caretakers. Suppose we were to utilize our own reactions as a teaching tool for modeling the best anxiety-management techniques. It can be good for our children's overall well-being and the self-care of parents. Modeling appropriate self-care, positive thinking, and anxiety approach behaviors can help youngsters cope with their own fears and anxieties.

Following are some suggestions for you to be a positive role model for your adolescent:

- Try to follow through on what you have told your youngster to do. When you do not, children can and will notice!

- Maintain a positive mindset by thinking, acting, and speaking positively.

- To deal with obstacles or disagreements calmly and productively, use problem-solving abilities. Getting irritated and angry encourages your youngster to do the same when a problem occurs.

- Treat yourself with the love, care, and compassion you would give to a friend or family member.

These are some productive parental strategies to help your child leave his worries behind and enjoy his life.

Chapter 5: Fear Toolkit

As this chapter deals with fears and phobias, let me clarify the difference between the two. It will help you understand how severe the problem is.

Fear is a strong emotional reaction. A genuine or perceived threat might trigger a person's fear response. Fear can be beneficial if it aids in the avoidance of a potentially dangerous circumstance. Many things can cause you to acquire anxieties, including dogs and to fly in an airplane. When confronted with a fear, some persons produce a fear reaction (such as shaking or sweating).

Phobia is a fear of something that is not dangerous. Irrational worries are a term used to describe phobias. The reaction is so strong that it may impair your ability to function or complete daily tasks. Anxiety symptoms might be triggered just by thinking about the feared item. The severity of your phobia's impact on your life is measured by its impairment, ranging from minor to severe. Even though you are not face-to-face with the thing, you may have a terror response if you have a phobia. If you have a phobia of dogs, just thinking about one can cause you to tremble or sweat.

The following strategies can help your child grow out of excessive fear.

5.1 Talk about It

It is crucial to approach a child's fear of the dark with sympathy and understanding, just as you would with other concerns. Do not mock or disregard your child's sentiments, and do not become upset and irritated as a result. Accepting your kid's feelings as real and responding to them sympathetically is the first major step in helping them overcome their unreasonable fear.

Here are some ideas for fear of the dark, changeable for other fears:

- Request that they tell you about their fears and what makes them fearful.

- Demonstrate to your youngster that you understand but do not necessarily share their anxieties.

- Reassure children that they are safe; explain, e.g., monsters do not exist.

- Checking in the cabinet or beneath the bed to comfort your child may make you believe monsters are lurking there.

- If your child is scared of the dark due to the threat of burglars, showing them the security features of your home, such as locks, may be beneficial. However, when people are inside the house, never lock a deadlock since it may prevent escape in the event of some emergency.

- Ask your youngster about what might make them feel more secure. Make your own suggestions. Perhaps bringing a toy or comforter to bed would make them feel better.

- Determine whether their dread of the dark stems from other concerns. Some youngsters, for example, maybe scared of their parents divorcing or dying, and this fear is exacerbated when they are alone in the dark. Discuss these topics openly with your youngster.

Moreover, kids may understand what they are afraid of, but they do not necessarily know how to express it. Specific queries can be beneficial. For example, if a child is terrified of dogs, you could ask, "What makes dogs scary?" "Did a dog catch you off guard or knock you down?" "Do you have a pet dog that you're terrified of?" You will have a well-informed idea of how to help your child overcome her fears once you understand what she's scared of.

However, fears might be difficult for youngsters to express. When confronted with straightforward inquiries, they become defensive. Children often open up more easily when creating characters with dolls or puppets. Perhaps it will be beneficial to your youngster.

Introduce a character who shares your child's fear when you are playing make-believe. Keep an eye on how your child's character reacts. Their response may reveal how your child is experiencing or how you might assist them. For example, if your youngster is scared of the dark, imagine that a puppet is as well. What is the reaction of your child's puppet? Does he ask you to close the bedroom drapes every night? Perhaps your youngster finds something similar to comfort him at night. Ask him. Even if your youngster says no, you have opened the lines of communication.

5.2 Validate Fears

Once you have figured out your child's worry, let him know you are taking it and him seriously. When a child describes something as frightening, we, as adults, do not agree most of the time. However, we must always begin by validating their feelings. Instead of saying things like "Oh, come on, that wasn't scary!" or "What is there to be afraid of?" say things like "Wow, that sounds like you were scared!" or "I know a lot of children are scared of that."

Validate your child's feelings, but do not overreact to his or her fear. If you pick up your fearful youngster every time he or she cries, you may unintentionally signal that there is something to be scared of. It could also mean that the only place you can feel safe is in your arms. Their favorite place is in your arms, but make the hug a reward for brave behavior rather than an unintended one for avoidant behavior. Rather than being overly reassuring, gently discuss what you see with them: 'That balloon startled you when it popped, didn't it?'

Lastly, it is critical to move on soon after providing reassurance. We do not want to focus on providing comfort in the face of the frightening situation since that, too, can become reinforcing and take on a life of its own. Instead, start talking about how you will help him feel braver and eventually be able to manage his fear on his own.

5.3 Fill in the Gaps

Younger children are still learning how to navigate the world. They are learning about cause and effect, and the fact that the result follows the cause is not always evident to newcomers. It may seem obvious that playing near a vacuum cleaner does not imply you will vanish into the end when it gets too close, but it is not so evident to a small child. Demonstrate how it works. A shoe, a foot, a chair, a vehicle, or a person will all fit into the vacuum's end, but a shoe, chair, foot, car, or a person will not. Even for older children – for anyone – the more information (numbers, facts) they have, the less concerned they will be. If they are afraid of thunderstorms, explain where thunder and lightning come from. Provide them with as much information as they require in order to feel protected.

5.4 Respect their Change of Mind

Once, while having my child's birthday party, a four-year-old girl was ecstatic to have her face painted in clown makeup. As she witnessed others transform into colorful clowns, she wriggled and giggled. Finally, I painted her face for her and showed her the mirror.

Then, all of a sudden, tears poured in. "I disappeared!" she screamed. "Take it off! Take it off!"

She changed her mind; the make-up had taken her identity, and she was terrified.

I could have said, "Don't be silly," You asked for it, so quit being stupid and have some fun with the other kids." What would there be any value in dismissing her feelings? Why should you deny her the right to change her mind? There are different ways to pretend that you are a clown.

She might like the make-up someday. But that day, I quickly removed the paint from her innocent face because it was hers to keep.

We often deny children the right to change their opinions. Kids love Santa or the Easter Bunny etc. But when they get face to face with the enormous stranger, they realize it is not such a good idea. Despite this, their parents encourage them to continue. We need to offer kids more decision-making power if we truly want them to appreciate experiences. It is sometimes best to let them change their mind.

It teaches kids to believe in their own judgment and gut feelings. They will overcome their fears in some time.

5.5 Make a Trigger List

In this part, we can clarify the triggers before making a plan to deal with them. Make a list of the situations or things your child is afraid of with your help. Go over the worst-case scenario with your youngster.

Similar fears can be grouped. For example, children who are scared that something awful will happen to their parents while they are separated may be afraid to go to school or someone else's house. They may be concerned about being left with a babysitter. All of these things are a component of the larger fear of being separated from you.

5.6 Take Little Steps

Set sensible goals with your youngster. Anxious children will frequently go to great lengths to avoid their anxieties. Unfortunately, avoiding them simply makes them more anxious. Although it may be frightening at first, confronting anxieties will help you overcome anxiety in the long term.

If your kid is scared of something specific, such as sleeping alone in the dark or meeting new people, use the stepladder approach to help them face their anxieties one small step at a time. The idea of this strategy is for them to perform something reasonably scary — and then practice it until it becomes less scary. They can then proceed to the next step.

However, it is critical to advance slowly. If you force your child to do something too frightening for them, they may become even more afraid, and your attempts will backfire.

Make a list with your kid of the measures they can take to tackle their fears and achieve their overall objective. If your kid insists on sleeping in your bed, here's an example of how you might assist them in overcoming their fear of sleeping alone:

- Place a mattress on the floor next to your bed for your child to sleep on.

- Place a mattress on the floor near the door, away from your bed, for your youngster to sleep on.

- Allow your child to sleep on a mattress on the floor in your room, with the understanding that after they fall asleep, you will place them in their own bed.

- Allow your child to fall asleep in their own room with you present.

- Allow your child to fall asleep in their own room with the understanding that you will check on them every few minutes till they fall asleep.

- Allow your youngster to fall asleep with the light on in their own room.

- Allow your youngster to sleep with only a nightlight in their own room.

For someone who is afraid of dogs, consider the following steps:

- Start with a dog-related book. Take some time to look at dog pictures.

- Switch to a cuddly toy dog. Touch it and hold it in your hands.

- Watch a film about a loving puppy.

- Hold a tiny, friendly dog in front of them and encourage them to look at it.

- Hold a little dog in your arms and urge them to pet it.

- Allow them to touch a small dog.

- Encourage them to look at a larger, friendlier dog.

- Encourage them to pat the larger friendly dog.

You might give your child extra privilege or an incentive if they reach a certain milestone. Natural consequences can also be used to motivate your youngster. If they are too bashful to order their own ice cream, you may tell them that they must do it if they want one. Of course, you should only use this if you are confident in their ability to accomplish it on their own.

You may have a few steps or a lot, depending on your child's phobia. However, it is critical to enlist your child's help at this time to ensure she's invested in making a difference.

5.7 Regulate Scary Media Consumption

Images from video games, movies, the internet, music videos, and late-breaking news articles can either provoke or exacerbate concerns. So keep an eye on your child's media intake, especially as sleep approaches.

Even better, teach your child to use the remote to turn off whatever is bothering him. "This is terrifying." "I do not need to watch it" is an excellent line for children to learn.

Assist your child in learning what types of movies are more soothing and fear-reducing. Have a pair of fun "giggle-producer" DVDs on hand for kids to watch when their anxiety levels rise. This will teach your children how to keep track of their own media consumption.

5.8 Communicate What to Expect

We cannot protect our children from all worries, and they must learn to live with them. Educating your youngster about the incident might help to dispel misconceptions and increase security.

If your youngster is concerned about "getting Corona-19," explain how you are following CDC (Centers for Disease Control and Prevention) standards. Discuss the CDC's suggestions with your child after seeing their website. "How can we keep ourselves secure at home?"

Keep your tone calm and matter-of-fact. "Would you like to talk about what your school is doing to keep you safe?" you might ask first. Visit your child's website to reassure him that a plan is in place (after you've double-checked that one is). Describe how the entire community, including the mayor, police, fire department, and doctors, is aware of the situation and will assist.

But what about anxiety causing upcoming events? Here is how you can help your little one feel more at ease about an impending hospital visit by letting him know what to expect: You may take him to the hospital, read books to talk about his anxieties, purchase him a toy doctor's kit to play with, and tell him to put his teddy bear and blanket into his backpack before he leaves.

Knowing what to expect – or realizing that the youngster has a safety plan that they practice and rehearse – might help alleviate that dread. Rehearse!

5.9 Rewire the Association

The issue with intense anxieties is that they get coupled with strong sentiments and memories — negative ones. Re-establish this link by associating something enjoyable or soothing with whatever is causing the problem. Children who are terrified of thunderstorms are one example of where this could be useful. If your child is afraid during a thunderstorm, acknowledge their fear and assure them that it is normal. Realize what they are feeling first (they need to know you are paying attention), then refocus - suggest watching a hilarious movie with him or her or coloring while listening to soothing music, even if it is through headphones. When they are ready, you can work up to a game — every time there is lightning, someone has to deliver a humorous joke (have lots prepared), and everyone eats m&m's till the thunder cracks – or something like that. Anything that shifts their attention away from their frightening ideas, memories, or sensations and onto something nice will assist in fading the bad associations.

5.10 Show Relaxation Strategies

If your child is tense as a result of the fear, learning relaxation techniques may help them regain control. Repeat the one tip until it is virtually "automatic." A pictorial reminder on the fridge or near your child's bed can be necessary. The idea is for your youngster to adopt that method as soon as the fear appears, rather than letting it build up. Here are a few suggestions:

- **Float Around:** Assume you are floating. "Imagine you are drifting peacefully on a cloud or lying quietly on a beach."

- **Lemon:** Muscle tension is relieved with this relaxing practice. Assume you are holding a lemon in your hand.

  - ➤ With each hand, reach up to the tree and pluck a lemon.

  - ➤ Squeeze the lemons vigorously to extract all of the juice - squeeze, squeeze, and squeeze.

  - ➤ Toss the lemons on the floor and take a deep breath.

  - ➤ Then do it again until you have got enough lemon juice to make a glass of lemonade!

  - ➤ Shake out your hands to relax after your last squeeze and toss!

- **Feather/Statue**: For around ten seconds, imagine yourself as a feather floating through the air.

  - ➤ You suddenly stop moving and turn into a statue. Do not move!

  - ➤ Then, when you convert back into the floating feather, relax.

  - ➤ Repeat, ensuring that you end up with an airy feather in a calm condition.

- **Lazy Cat**

  - ➤ Pretend you are a sleepy cat who has just awoken from a long snooze.

> Have a large yawn and a meow.

> Now slowly stretch your limbs, legs, and back, as if you were a cat, and relax.

- **Turtle**
  > Pretend you are a turtle taking a calm, relaxing stroll.
  > It is starting to rain, oh no! For around ten seconds, curl up tight under your shell.
  > Come out of your shell and resume your peaceful walk now that the sun has returned.
  > Rep a few times more, finishing with a walk to ensure your body is relaxed.
- **Stress Balls**

This practice relaxes your muscles while massaging your hands.

> Fill balloons with dry lentils or rice to make your own stress ball(s).

> Squeeze and release the ball(s) in one or both hands.

> Squeeze the ball and see what happens. Find a way that works for you by altering your squeezes' speed, pressure, and timing to your liking.

5.11 Teach Self-Assuring Talk

Help your child learn to overcome her fears by teaching her positive statements. It is best to assist your child in picking just one word and asking her to repeat it several times a day until she can say it to herself when she is feeling anxious. Ask to gently and lovingly deliver these statements. For example, "I can do this," "This is not going to be a problem for me." or "I'll be OK."

The power of affirmations comes from their uplifting aspect, but we also want them to be credible! Instead of "wishful thinking," children should use affirmations to remind themselves of their inherent strength and abilities, which concern might exploit. Here are some more statements:

- **I am safe.**

  This is a powerful affirmation to remind youngsters of the reality of the situation when they are genuinely in a safe place. Combine it with grounding practices to help children become more aware of their surroundings.

- **My breathing is under my control.**

  Things can feel out of hand at times. With this affirmation, kids may remember that they can manage their own breathing to relax their bodies.

- **I can try.**

  This is an excellent encouragement for youngsters who are afraid of failing or making mistakes and are hesitant to begin projects or try new things.

- **I can tell my fears to go away.**

  Help kids become more aware of their skills to personify fears and take control of their anxiety! Kids can tell their fear that it is wrong, that it should leave, and that they have had enough of listening to it.

- **It may be difficult, but I am capable of handling it.**

  With this affirmation, kids can learn to tap into their inner strength.

5.12 Encourage Realistic Thinking

It is easier to believe the worst will happen when you are afraid. It is the brain's attempt to keep us safe from harm. This is something you can tell your youngster. You might also explain to your child that the brain is not always sure whether or not the risk is real.

Encourage your kid to be a "thinking detective." Have your youngster do the following:

- Pay attention to the following ideas: "If Mom goes to the grocery store without me, she'll get hurt," your youngster may believe.

- Determine whether it is a fact or a feeling: Rephrase the preceding thinking as "I'm concerned that Mom will get wounded if I am not with her at the grocery shop."

- Gather evidence to support or refute it: When Mom went to the supermarket alone before, she was fine when she returned home.

- Challenge the idea: Some children can learn to "argue" with themselves, arguing both sides and convincing themselves that the idea is incorrect.

5.13 Avoid Avoiding Fear

When children exhibit extreme anxiety or fear, it is logical that a caring parent would desire to shield them from these negative emotions. It can feel as if the only way to relieve their pain is to support their avoidance, whether it is due to weariness or a lack of options. This can provide everyone with short-term respite (which is often badly needed), but avoidance has a sneaky way of making the situation worse ultimately and feeding anxiety.

Avoidance deprives children of the opportunity to learn that whatever is concerning them is unlikely to occur and that if it does, they are strong, resilient, and resourceful enough to deal with it. Fear is a warning, not a prediction, and there is no way to learn this. Instead, children learn that avoiding an odd or unpleasant circumstance is the best way to deal with it. The more something is kept at arm's length, the more confirmed it is that the best way to stay safe is to avoid it Avoidance may be a smart decision at times, but it may also impede their ability to reach out into the world.

Our brains are always evolving to become the best brain possible for us. It accomplishes this through personal experience. The brain strengthens the corresponding connections when an experience is repeated. It will alter itself in response to what it believes we require, and this will be based on our repeated behaviors. If avoidance is a habitual response, the brain will adapt to accommodate it. The good news is that, just as the brain changes itself without our conscious effort, we can change it in ways that are more in line with our needs by intentionally exposing the brain to particular experiences. It is called experience-dependent neuroplasticity, and it affects everyone, including children.

5.14 Teach Self-Regulation

So, how can we encourage little ones to become braver? Self-regulation, an intangible talent, is the key. The skill to understand and manage your own emotions and behaviors healthily is known as self-regulation. It is what allows us to talk ourselves down or sense emotions without acting on them. Self-regulation is something that most adults do without thinking about it. Consider experiencing a brief moment of terror before telling yourself that a dark room is nothing to be afraid of. On the other hand, building self-regulation in children takes time, experience, and room to learn – which means parents must become comfortable with letting their children be a little uncomfortable while they figure things out.

Remember that children are in survival mode when they react at the moment. Their lower brains are working overtime. Do not attempt to reason with them because they cannot respond to logic. Instead, remain cool, empathize with them, assist them in being self-aware, and lead them through sensory experiences and calming techniques.

Assist them in comprehending the role of the downstairs brain in stress reaction and the role of the upstairs brain in control. Improve their vocabulary. Talk to your kids about their emotions.

Improve their self-awareness to aid in self-monitoring. Allow youngsters to rank their emotions and energy reserves on a scale of 1 to 5. Assist them in identifying calming tactics and ways to replenish their resource pool.

Refrain from punishing uncontrollable behavior. Rather, utilize it as a beginning point for determining where youngsters require assistance. Remember that punishing children will not teach them the skills they need to regulate their emotions.

Ensure that the children's resource pool for regulation is supplied regularly. A healthy diet, sleep, and regular exercise are all important. Assist youngsters in making plans for activities they enjoy and excel in.

5.15 Give Your Child Control

According to studies, having a sense of control over a situation helps to reduce anxiety. As a result, empower your child by assisting him in developing his own fear-reduction strategy. Start by tackling a single fear.

"The strange shadows on my wall make me afraid to sleep in the dark," says the problem.

"What could make you feel safer?" says the parent. Then brainstorm plausible possibilities with your child until he can come up with at least one that will help him feel more in control, and then put it into action.

"Shift my bed away from the bookcase, so I do not see the shadows on the wall," a child may suggest.

I hope these strategies help your child overcome his fears. Our world is unpredictable and uncertain. We cannot protect our children from what life offers, no matter how hard we try. However, we can assist our children in learning to handle their worries and anxiety. We can also teach our children coping methods to aid their development of the agency. Children who have a "We've Got This" attitude toward life are more likely to succeed. They will employ those coping methods to assist them in dealing with whatever adversity they face and increase their overall resilience.

Chapter 6: Insecurity Toolkit

When a kid is insecure within himself, he is automatically insecure around others. This chapter will discuss parental strategies for helping children be more confident about themselves and strategies for the many other factors contributing to social anxiety.

Children with a social anxiety disorder (SAD) may experience symptoms far into adulthood before being diagnosed. Many parents are unmindful of the symptoms of SAD in children and teenagers, even though it is the third most occurring mental health disorder.

A strong fear or phobia of performance and social situations characterizes social anxiety disorder. Kids with social anxiety disorder are nervous in various situations, not just at parties or when giving a speech in class. It is actually not a fear of being in social situations; it is a fear of how people perceive you.

Small interactions, such as answering a question in class or having lunch with friends in the cafeteria, can be terrifying for children with social anxiety disorder. This is because they are afraid of doing something embarrassing or insulting by accident, which may cause others to condemn or reject them.

And, unlike timid children who warm up to new people and settings with time, children with social anxiety do not. Now let's move towards the solution.

6.1 Connect and Understand

Would it not be incredible if you could figure out why your child has insecurities and help them deal with them so they do not have to struggle for the rest of their adult lives? When you see your child teetering on the edge of an overwhelming self-doubt precipice, go in and save them.

The most powerful impact on children is that of their parents. Not only will figuring out the "why" enrich your bond with your child, but it will also provide you with insight into how to help them navigate through life's challenges.

The PACE concept can engage your children and make them feel comfortable. PACE stands for Playfulness, Acceptance, Curiosity, and Empathy. By letting the youngster know that you are relaxed and able to understand and support them, these four reactions or styles of interaction serve to relieve some of the anxiety connected with a scenario.

- **Playfulness** demonstrates to your child that you, the person who keeps them safe, are relaxed and open, allowing them to relax.

  "You appear to be concerned about your upcoming game. Are you concerned that you'll have too much fun?"

- **Accepting** your child's feelings is especially crucial if your child has anxiety because worry is frequently dismissed as illogical. Your child will feel safer now and in the future if they learn that they can come to you with their anxiety and be heard.

"Perhaps you're concerned about missing a goal the next day. When I focus on scoring in sports, I know I experience a lot of anxiety and pressure to do well. I am curious if you are concerned because you are unsure if you will meet your goals."

- To help draw out what the child is feeling, introduce a **curiosity** about the child's feelings. Sometimes the child feels understood right away. However, if you are wrong, your youngster may reveal what they are really worried about.

"Well, I did miss a goal in the last game, and Jordan was upset with me because I let the entire team down."

"That is extremely difficult! It's a huge, weighty feeling to feel like you've let the whole squad down."

- **Empathizing** with the child's sentiments allows them to feel more connected to you since you understand how they are feeling rather than just what they are saying.

This paradigm allows the child to feel heard and connected, two qualities that might help the youngster cope in stressful situations. You can work on ways to manage your child's social anxiety after they are interacting with you in a safe and empathic environment.

6.2 Teach them Self-Love

Contrary to popular assumptions, self-love is about appreciating both the positive and bad aspects of oneself. It is about learning to understand that our flaws are a part of who we are and work on them to evolve. It is also about learning to love every aspect of ourselves - big, tiny, and everything in between – and prioritizing our needs over pleasing others.

- Knowing that they are respected and appreciated does wonders for your children's self-esteem. Allow them to participate in day-to-day activities to make them feel significant. Making decisions, accompanying you on supermarket runs, or even allowing them to assist you with your job can give them the sense that their presence and ideas are valued. They will want to come forward gladly in the future to take on tasks that they believe they can overcome.

- Kids sometimes need to be prompted to evaluate themselves and determine how they feel about their accomplishments and setbacks. "How do you feel about winning this game?" you might ask. This will reinforce the idea that happiness comes from within, not from others' approval. It provides a channel for people to express their feelings. As kids get more interested in expressing themselves, they will begin to feel closer to themselves and to you. Show children how to reward themselves by doing something they enjoy, even if it is not for a specific reason. Exercise self-reflection with them to see what ticks them off. This is how kids will learn in the future to pay careful attention to their mental health.

- How many times have you told a youngster, "Aww, you are such a strong/beautiful girl?" or "wow, you're such a strong/beautiful boy?" It is something we have all done. On the other hand, surface-level compliments can do more harm than good to a child's self-esteem. Complimenting your child's intellect and rewarding good attempts (rather than just good results) will boost their self-esteem in ways you cannot conceive.

They would not value themselves based on grades if you tell them an A is excellent and a C is a terrific attempt. At the same time, they will most likely put in more effort to get an A. Compliments play an important role in the lives of children. They serve as a form of reinforcement, assuring them that certain behaviors are appropriate and respectable. So, compliment them, but do so in a proper manner.

- Most essential, let them know that self-love is not linear. It is a tough thing to accept. Tell your children that self-love takes time, practice, and progress. It is not a guarantee of happiness for the rest of your life. The truth is that it is a work in progress and a journey. Remind your kids that they may not always love themselves and may even feel lost. However, emphasize that feeling this way is normal and human. What matters is that they learn to pick themselves up and move forward. Teach them to comfort themselves in this way: "Today, I do not love myself." But tomorrow is a fresh day, so I will give it another shot."

Here's a self-love fun activity for your child:

"' I Love Myself' Jar" is a fantastic way to teach your youngster to appreciate themselves! Have your children write down something they like about themselves on a sheet of paper every day. If they are not in the mood for self-love on that particular day, they can opt for something more neutral. After that, place it in a jar. This jar may be decorated; however, they would want to make it fun and memorable for them to enjoy. You can open up the jar at the end of each week or every two weeks (you pick) and read the nice things your kids wrote about themselves.

They not only reinforce their self-image every day, but they also receive a love jackpot when they read all of their letters at once! They are reminded of why they are so special and why they should cherish themselves every day! They will eventually learn to hold on to those messages and keep them inside as they navigate a world that tells them they are not good enough the way they are.

6.3 Equip them with Knowledge

One of the most fruitful techniques you can apply is to provide your youngster with as much information about some event as possible. Consider the location, who will be present, and what might happen. Scripting, role-playing, and previewing are all useful strategies for the socially anxious child.

Kathy Radigan's son, now a college freshman, was speech delayed as a child, which made him fearful of meeting new people. Radigan says, "But he wanted to play with kids."

"To assist him in getting past those first few nervous moments, we used scripting." "We would do some role-playing," she continues. "I'd tell him about a boy who went to the park and became worried when he saw the kids," I said.

Radigan's son performed small scripts with her, such as "Hello, Tom." "What are your favorite games to play?" She claims it was generally sufficient to break the ice. Her son recalls that those early years of scripting and role-playing were quite beneficial.

Role-playing and previewing make the activity feel less unfamiliar and terrifying, so the youngster is less likely to be overwhelmed when time comes for the real event. Although not everything can be predicted, having a rough idea can make children feel a lot more at ease.

6.4 Take Baby Steps

It is unrealistic to expect children who are anxious in social situations to be able to jump straight in. Arriving early or late may assist them, and they will need to adjust at their own rate. Many people will prefer to observe for a time before getting involved.

For example, you can help your child negotiate the experience on her own terms by providing her time and permission. You can encourage her to take small steps out of her comfort zone, such as starting by watching the other children, then coming closer, then playing near them, and finally playing with them.

Another effective strategy is to arrive early to check out the situation. If you are going to a new group or activity, arriving fifteen minutes early can help them relax and appreciate the area without the bustle of other children.

Of course, every effort is deserving of applause, whether it is sitting on the edge of a party or completely engaged. It could be as easy as, "I appreciate how you came over and sat down to have a slice of pizza." This is a far better strategy than engaging in a power battle over why they are not having fun.

When getting your child "on stage," think of less stressful ways. An example would be asking the teacher to send home a question so that your child can practice answering it before speaking in class. Request permission to record a video of your child's report at home, or perhaps stage a puppet show from behind a curtain.

6.5 Teach Cognitive Reframing

Negative beliefs that encourage anxious thinking can overwhelm children with social anxiety disorder. Their beliefs are generally divided into the groups below:

- Believing that others have a negative perspective of them

- Assuming the worst-case scenario

- Personalizing

- Overreacting

Teach your youngster to notice and replace bad thoughts with positive thoughts. If your little one says things like, "My teacher thinks I'm stupid because I can't read," help him point out the negative thought, give it a reality check (a teacher's job is to help students learn, not to judge them based on what they already know), and change it with a new and positive thought ("I'm having trouble reading, but I will get better with my teacher's help.")

Let's study some strategies for cognitive distortions:

- **What-Ifs**

  What if I throw up? What if I fail the exam? What if I get sick? What if they do not like me? What ifs abound in the minds of anxious children. We tell them that these "terrible" things aren't going to happen most of the time to help them relax.

  But is this helpful? Acceptance is a better, less intuitive technique to help our children deal with some anxiety issues.

  What is the worst that can happen if you throw up? What are your options for dealing with that? What is the worst that can happen if you fail a test? What are your options for dealing with that?

  When we have transition from reassurance to problem-solving, it is quite effective. When a youngster already has a plan to deal with the "worst-case scenario," they can feel empowered. Even just imagining what might happen and how they would manage it might help to alleviate anxiety.

- **The Negative Filter**

  A very difficult moment for parents is to find their little one criticizing himself or making remarks like, "I can't do this because I'm stupid," or "He won't play with me and be my friend because I'm stupid." These remarks, which are linked to poor self-esteem, are extremely harmful. Without due attention, they can significantly impact a child's self-esteem.

When your child claims she is "dumb," "stupid," or "worthless," it is natural as a parent to become so emotionally invested in her pain that you have trouble hearing her rationally. You need to consider how you would react if you were in your child's situation. Is it possible that his self-perception is linked to his ability to solve a math problem or connection with his peers?

You can help your youngster determine WHAT is upsetting him and start to isolate the issue from his own self-worth if you can find out what he is feeling and name it.

For example, you can separate the problem from the self-worth in the statement "He won't be my friend because I am stupid" in the following ways:

Ask him, "Why do you think you are stupid?" Whatever answer he gives you is the problem, and you can help him find solutions for it.

If your child does not respond clearly and you feel it is because he lacks confidence or social skills, you can help him work it out.

Moreover, you can demonstrate that the issue as a whole is not frustrating, but only a part of it like:

1. "Up to this point, your numbers appear to be fantastic. Is this when things start to get more difficult?"

2. "Could you tell me at what point your math homework starts to get tricky?"

- **Blowing out of Proportion**

  Pay attention to your child and take in what they have to say. Rephrase or repeat what was said. "I'll never win the prize," for example, can be rephrased as "It seems like things are not going your way."

  Take the belief and replace it with hope or an alternative. Avoid opposite statements like "Yes, you will; you are clever." Make an effort to understand your child's feelings and gently help them to see other perspectives. For example, "I understand that you are concerned about how you will perform on the test. Can I do anything to make you feel better?"

  Remember to listen to your child. You will encounter resistance if you abruptly dismiss a remark or sensation.

  Meet your little one in the mental state he is right now. Assist them in easing into a less severe position. You want your youngster to get there on their own and adjust their mindset to "Maybe I'll win if I share my ideas" rather than "Maybe I'll lose if I share my ideas."

- **Everything is Personal**

  Your child must not let negative remarks dictate how he sees himself because they are mostly wrong. "When you go into a room, no one is thinking of you; they think of themselves," goes an old proverb. It means that when people look at you and judge you, they are doing it in light of their feelings. Their viewpoint is biased in their favor. And that is exactly what my strategy is based on: exposing the fact that it is just one person's biased viewpoint. "It is not you. It is them." It reflects on the other person in the same way that your own behaviors do.

You want your youngster to be self-assured. Respect himself. Take responsibility for his actions, not of others.

6.6 Develop Friendship Skills

However, you may assist your child in honing his or her social skills by providing opportunities to practice new ones. Make use of role-playing and role-modeling to help your youngster feel more at ease around others:

- Greetings

- Moving in and out of groups.

- Starters for the conversation

- listening and responding

- Following up by additional questions or making additional statements

At times, it can be as simple as finding common ground or arriving with someone with whom your child is already at ease. Children, like most people, are more comfortable entering new social situations with a partner.

"Sometimes, I ease the transition in a larger group by introducing him to someone," says Dawn Alicot of her six-year-old. I am on the lookout for common ground." For example, it can be spotting a kid wearing the same sneakers or a favorite cartoon character's shirt. Alicot reports that her son began doing this on his own after some time and has successfully made friends in this manner.

6.7 Make Plans for In and Out of Class

Carpooling is a great way to get your youngster to a party or new karate class with a friend. Ask your child's teacher to pair him or her with a friendly classmate who can answer questions about what to bring and what to wear for school projects. Having a friend along for the ride might lessen the stress of social situations.

Plan for lunch and break times. Youngsters have the freedom to make their own rules when there is no set schedule. There is a good chance that your child will have difficulty interpreting the signals in his or her environment. Use these less structured times of the day, work with school staff and teachers to help your child deal with social anxiety. This cannot be left to chance. Your child is more likely to fail than succeed if he does not have a strategy.

6.8 Monitor their Social Media

Social media can be a major factor in your child's sense of insecurity, especially in this day and age of digital domination. Especially trolls, harsh comments, or unfavorable judgments can impact your child. As a result, they stay up to date on their social and personal activities. Do not, however, intrude on their privacy or cause them distress.

6.9 Focus on Progress

Perfectionism and social anxiety are closely connected. A child's nervous sentiments are exacerbated by the fear of failing, looking bad in front of friends, or the dread of not meeting a goal.

Encourage your child to place more emphasis on the journey than the destination. Talk about how much you like hearing them practice the flute and how much fun it is to play sports with them.

This is an amazing opportunity to reaffirm your understanding of the growth mindset and the importance of making mistakes. Rather than bragging about your accomplishments, share your failures and the lessons you have learned in your journey.

Use the phrase "Practice IS the goal" as a guideline in your daily life. Statements like "finding comfort in the practice" and "enjoying the trip" have real significance in reminding us to enjoy the process rather than obsess over the result.

When your kids follow this mindset, their happiness is not only confined to the few minutes they feel when they achieve a goal; it lasts far longer. Instead, they are ecstatic about the entire process since they can see their development and take pleasure in it.

6.10 Boundaries and Aches

It is essential to remember that your child's physical complaints may be an attempt to shield him from something he finds frightening. Ask for specifics so that you can assist your child in developing a plan of action. "Can I do something to make it better?"

It is time to draw some clear lines. For example, "You can't miss school unless you have a fever," "You can have 15 minutes of break, then you need to get back to doing the work." Having your youngster rate the difficulty of the task might also be helpful. You will be able to tell if your youngster is resisting because he or she believes the task is too difficult.

6.11 Stop Comparing

When we want to help our children succeed, it is easy to cave into the temptation to compare. "Do you see how well Elise manages her rage?" "Cannot you do that?" "Ray isn't so shy. You could be like him if you tried a bit harder."

We are sending our child the message, "I like that child over you."

Studies have shown that youngsters who are commended for being better at something than someone else only keep their motivation going as long as they keep winning and getting praised. To avoid losing, they quickly learn to avoid taking chances. Their primary focus shifts to staying competitive and getting recognition from their peers. Insecure children are more likely to develop jealousy when others receive praise from you.

However, mastery-based praise, which encourages a child's efforts and accomplishments, is a wonderful antidote to insecurity and envy. It builds intrinsic motivation and a healthy feeling of self-worth.

6.12 Focus on Your Relationship

I put love notes in my kid's lunchboxes. I would sketch or paint a comical face or picture on a hard-boiled egg to cheer them up. Your egg-ceptional! All the best for this new day! To say, "I love you just because" was the intent of these words. I put encouragement notes on their bedroom doors.

You can paste sticky notes on the mirror where children get ready for school. For example,

"You have my utmost admiration and devotion." "You are in my thoughts today." "I have faith in you." Be thankful for them and the relationship you have with them.

Children's feelings about themselves are quickly influenced by their messages about themselves from others. Harsh statements ("You're so lazy!") are dispiriting rather than motivating. Children's self-esteem is damaged when you say negative things about them. Patience is key while addressing children. Concentrate on what you would like them to do the next time. Show them how to do it if necessary.

Children who know that they are loved unconditionally by their parents, regardless of how well they perform, are more comfortable when their parents praise other children. They understand that their worth is not tied to their ability to outperform others.

6.13 Know When to Step Back

It is a bit more complicated because it depends on the child. Parents who hover over their worried children can actually increase their own anxiety since they can sense the parent's concern. Take a step back, but keep an eye on them if they need your help.

To help your child cope with an impending panic attack or episode, you can remove them from the situation for a short period to practice their self-calming techniques like deep breathing and mindfulness and then return. This is a logical step. You are the person who truly understands your child. Even though it is terrifying, allow your child to explore and grow, even if it is uncomfortable.

These strategies can help a child grow confidence and be secure around others.

Chapter 7: Stress Toolkit

As providers and caregivers, adults tend to see children's world as cheerful and carefree. After all, kids do not have to worry about keeping their jobs or paying their bills, so what could they possibly be worried about?

Plenty! Even the tiniest youngsters worry and are stressed in some way.

According to a national WebMD study, parents report the main sources of stress in their children's life as school and friends. According to the report, 72 percent of children exhibit bad behaviors, and 62 percent have bodily symptoms such as stomachaches and headaches due to stress.

The activation of the stress response system for a long time and the subsequent overexposure to cortisol and other stress hormones can badly affect your body's systems. This puts kids at risk for anxiety and depression, among other health issues.

So how can we help children cope with stress?

7.1 Reframe Stress

Help your child change his mentality from "stress hurts" to "stress helps." If youngsters understand that unpleasant conditions will not persist forever, stress can be a catalyst for growth. Instead, these events serve as obstacles to be overcome and lessons to be learned.

Ian Robertson, a cognitive neuroscientist, and author compares the stress response system to the immune system: with practice, it becomes more powerful.

After a significant stress response, the brain rewires itself to remember and learn from the experience. This is how your brain trains you to deal with similar stressful events in the future.

The brain secretes the chemical noradrenaline in response to stress. When the brain has too much noradrenaline, it cannot function properly. It is also not good to have too little noradrenaline.

According to Robertson, reasonable stress levels can actually strengthen brain function, making individuals smarter and happier.

To get started, follow the steps below:

Adopt the "stress reliever" mentality. You need to accept that you would not be able to avoid stress as some stress is beneficial, and that stress can be a learning opportunity. It will be nearly impossible to teach this mindset to your child if you do not have it yourself. Plus, stress can be "contagious," so lowering your own is essential. When your child senses your stress, their physiology changes, and they go into stress mode.

Rather than dismissing your child's tension, try to figure out what is causing it. A child's troubles may appear insignificant to an adult. However, they appear to be large to the child, causing genuine stress or discomfort to the child.

Talk about the following points with your child to help him reframe stress:

- Stress is an unavoidable component of everyday living.

- Stress is not permanent.

- If you learn from stressful situations, take action, and seek solutions, they can benefit. Give specific instances from your own life.

Assist your child in identifying areas of development or lessons that can be learned from their most recent challenge.

- Request your youngster to recall any previous stressful situations. What did they take away from such encounters?

- What skills did they employ to deal with these situations?

- What strengths do they have right now?

Your youngster will establish a much healthier connection with stress and find it simpler to manage once it is perceived as an opportunity for growth.

7.2 Change Fixed Mindset to Growth Mindset

You and your youngster need a shift from a fixed to a growth perspective. According to studies, even quick growth mindset training decreases stress and improves grades in children.

We often feel overwhelmed in difficult situations and are more inclined to fall into a fixed mindset thought process, believing that there is nothing we can do to change the situation. We believe that our abilities are restricted to what we can achieve and that we should give up.

For example, if your youngster is worried about tests, they may believe, "It doesn't matter how much I study. I will never pass these tests. It's a hopeless situation."

Encourage your child to view the situation through the lens of a growth mindset: it is not fixed, it can be better, and they do have the ability to change it.

If you hear your child say something fixed mentality like "I can't do this" or "I'm just not good at math," encourage them to switch to a growth mindset.

Encourage your child to use growth mindset affirmations, and remind them that putting out effort and experimenting with new ideas will help them solve the problem and lessen stress.

7.3 Putting a Stop on Catastrophic Thinking

Anxiety and stress in youngsters can manifest in children as catastrophic thinking. It happens when a person anticipates the worst in everyday events. For example, a youngster may be apprehensive about going to school on the first day of class. Instead of experiencing regular anxiousness, he may outright refuse to attend school. When the lights go off, a youngster who is terrified of the dark may think something awful will happen to her. Therefore, she may stay awake as long as possible.

Breaking through the habits of catastrophic thinking that typically accompany anxiety problems in children may be stressful – and daunting – for parents. However, there are various strategies that parents may use to assist their children in refocusing their thoughts in more positive directions.

Parents may help their children with catastrophic thinking in three ways:

- **A Feelings Journal**

  Keeping the child's age and ability in mind, it is generally beneficial to keep a feelings diary (younger children may find it helpful to draw pictures instead.) Parents should urge their children to write down (or sketch) their worries whenever they occur. Journaling "feelings" allows the youngster to address sensations as they arise rather than bottling them up, prolonging anxious feelings and unpleasant ideas. This is a big step in figuring out what's causing your catastrophic thinking.

  Parents should then take this process further by discussing their emotions diary with their children. This is crucial to the child's capacity to recognize the sources of their catastrophic ideas. Children and their parents may take the next step in avoiding negative thoughts and, in some cases, eliminating them entirely by identifying triggers. Even if there are no identified triggers, children must talk about their feelings with an adult they can trust.

- **Catch It in the Act**

  Catching a youngster in the process of catastrophic thinking is one of the most effective methods to "reprogram" his negative thinking. It is critical for parents and other family members to be aware of the warning indications. For example, if a kid refuses to go to school, this is an apparent indicator of anxiety;

nevertheless, it is also vital to detect less evident signals of catastrophic thinking, like isolation or claims of physical symptoms. This is the time for the parent to have a conversation with the youngster about how he is feeling right now.

When anxious ideas occur, parents can encourage their children to approach them. An important element of this process is to assist the youngster in rationally processing these thoughts by questioning the kid. When children are experiencing thoughts of imminent disaster, parents might ask them the following questions:

> ➢ What triggered your thoughts?

> ➢ Do these thoughts make you feel worse or better?

> ➢ What are the chances that these ideas will become a reality?

Children will ultimately be able to adopt the positive self-talk necessary to extinguish or at least lessen these ideas on their own due to talking through these catastrophic thoughts. It is vital to remember that the catastrophic ideas that originate from worry are not reasonable; hence, teaching the youngster that their fears are unlikely to come true needs time and effort for long-term success. The ultimate objective is for youngsters to be able to catch themselves in the process of thinking and stop them before they spiral out of control.

- **Shift Focus**

  This is a simple yet powerful strategy for transforming negative thoughts into more positive ones. If your kids feel uncomfortable in social situations, refocus their attention, sing a jingle together or count how many people are wearing red shirts. Alternatively, talk about something they find interesting or an upcoming event — anything that will divert attention away from the negative thoughts.

It is essential to remember that consistency and patience are the keys to success with these tactics; do not expect to see results right away. Although there may likely be tiny indicators of success, modifying the mind's thinking is similar to remodeling the body. Progress must be achieved in manageable chunks, just as it must be accomplished in reasonable chunks while reshaping thinking. It is critical to acknowledge and recognize little achievements.

7.4 Teach Positive Self-Talk

Positive self-talk is a coping technique that aids in the development of positive thinking and self-esteem. It is a crucial aspect of social-emotional learning, and it has been found to boost positivity and help people gain self-confidence. Teaching children the importance of positive self-talk at a young age is also a terrific method to help them build resilience against challenges. Here's how you can do it:

- **Recognize the Negative Thought**

  Negative thoughts are often all-or-nothing claims that jump to conclusions. Certain words are red lights when it comes to negative self-talk. "I can't," "never," or "always" are words to keep an eye out for. For example,

  - ➢ "I never have fun since I'm not a good player!"

  - ➢ "I always look bad. I'm the slowest of them all!"

  Stop and talk to your children when they say things like this. Then you may assist them in thinking and saying more positive things instead.

- **Find Reasoning**

  To start, inquire as to why they said what they did. You might find they are fixated on something they have "messed up." Perhaps another child said something hurtful, such as "You are slow."

  Remind them that you love them. If another child said anything hurtful, attempt to put it in a context like:

  - ➢ "They must have had a rough day or do not feel good about themselves."

  - ➢ If they feel like they "failed," assure them that they will get another chance to try and excel at many things.

- **Re-assuring Statements**

  After that, have them mention something kind about themselves. They can tell themselves those positive and encouraging words whenever they undertake something new or challenging. These affirmative statements have the potential to boost one's self-esteem. For example, "I'm strong and a good teammate."

  He might say it every time he is going to walk onto the soccer field or when he is feeling apprehensive.

  If they do not succeed, you can teach them to put a positive spin on things.

  Reframe statements like "I messed up. I hate myself" to "The pass didn't work out the way I wanted. I'll work on my passing skills and try next game again."

- **Put in Practice**

  If your child is terrified of not being able to speak in front of her class, ask why she feels this way. Maybe she does not think she is prepared enough. Assure her that you believe she is capable of completing the task. Then assist her in practicing some more. Ask her to think of some good things she can say about herself when she is frightened or unhappy, such as "I practiced this." "I'll give my best."

- **Model It**

  It is vital to let your youngster hear you talking positively to yourself. Avoid saying things like "I can't,"

"I never," and "I always." Instead, model phrases like "I know today was difficult, but I can try again tomorrow" or "I believe I can be my best" that you want your child to say to herself.

7.5 Stop Overscheduling

Overscheduling is one of the biggest causes of stress for children. Despite this, today's children are expected to pay attention and do well in school for seven hours, succeed in extracurricular activities, return home, complete homework, and go to bed, just repeat the process the next day. "Where is the downtime?"

Downtime is necessary for children's rejuvenation. Their bodies and minds require rest. And it is possible that they are not aware of it. It is crucial to recognize when your youngster is overworked.

I recommend taking a week's worth of your kids' schedules and ensuring there's enough downtime — "when you're not monitoring the clock." Is there a time during the weekend or a few nights during the week when your youngster can just relax and unwind?

Pay attention to how your family eats their meals as well. Is everyone eating on the move, in the car, grab-and-go? That is a sign that there is a lot going on.

7.6 Teach Kids to Read their Body

Teach your children about their bodies and stress physiology. Sit in the car with your child and press the gas and brake pedals while listening to the motor rev. Our body just revs and revs until it wears out and says 'enough."

Motivate children to pay attention to their bodies' messages. While it is typical for a child's stomach to feel jittery on the first day of school waking up with a headache or leaving class because their stomach hurts regularly are signs that something is wrong.

You can help them understand how stress affects:

- Body (e.g., muscles that hurt, upset stomach, headache)

- Feelings (e.g., bad mood, irritability)

- Thoughts (e.g., difficulty paying attention, negative thoughts)

- Behavior (e.g., restlessness)

Continue to be a "stress detective" for younger children, assisting them in making connections between their bodies and stress. If you notice your child has a stomach ache or is more irritable than normal, and you suspect stress is to blame, you might encourage them to consider how their feelings may be related to stress. Remind them that stress is normal.

7.7 Help Name It

It takes time and practice to become aware of and identify your emotions. Children may not realize that the feelings they are experiencing are tied to a stressor.

Teach children the vocabulary to explain their emotions so they can express themselves to you. Giving feelings a name can be a huge comfort for kids. Younger children can be taught simple emotion terms such as happy, sad, mad, and scared. Older children can learn more complex feeling terms like frustrated, nervous, and disappointed. Feelings can be better managed by breaking them down.

7.8 Celebrate Little Wins

When confronted with a new issue, most children experience some anxiety. However, they eventually dive in because previous victories have given them confidence. Children who learn and think in various ways require the same drive, but the victories are sometimes more difficult. Keep an eye out for moments to congratulate them on a well-done job. Perhaps your child completed a few more word problems at the table without getting up. This is a victory! Knowing how to feel successful can help your youngster feel less overwhelmed when confronted with new problems.

7.9 Imperfect is Perfect

We often believe that our children's success in school, sports, and performance situations is required. However, we must remember that children must be allowed to be children. If an 85 is good but not good enough, school becomes driven by grades rather than enjoyment of learning. This is not to say that working hard is not necessary. It is crucial to encourage your child to work hard, but it is also critical to accept and cherish your child's flaws.

7.10 Teach Problem Solving

Before problem-solving becomes part of your child's routine, it will require a lot of examples, modeling, and real-world experience.

A smart place to start is to educate your child on the three-step method outlined below:

- The first step to take is to help him name and validate his emotions. Ask your child to describe how they are feeling, such as overwhelmed, worried, or anxious, and then repeat it back to them. "I understand you're concerned about your exam results."

- The second step is to deal with Emotions. Assist your youngster in finding their calming spot. It is good to make one if they do not already have one. Allow them to process their emotions and soothe their bodies so they can problem-solve, learn, and grow. You might have older kids practice deep breathing or growth mindset affirmations. "If I try, I can do well on this test."

- The last step is to solve the problem! Brainstorm solutions with your child, paying more attention to listening than speaking. For example, your child might come up with alternatives like studying with a buddy who is doing well in class, asking the teacher for extra help, or spending a set amount of time each day studying.

After you have come up with a few ideas, let your youngster consider the benefits and drawbacks of each one before deciding on one. Although your child may require encouragement, try to limit your contributions to open-ended questions, enabling your child to solve the majority of the problems independently.

If the first plan (let's call it Plan A) fails, your child will have a variety of backup plans ready to go. Knowing this will make their problem a lot easier to deal with. Youngsters will have the resources they need to deal with stressful situations on their own once they have mastered the art of problem-solving.

7.11 Energize the Body

Physical activity reduces stress hormone levels in the body while also increasing chemicals in the brain that improve mood and lessen pain. It has been demonstrated to improve well-being and quality of life while reducing symptoms of sadness and anxiety. Here are some ideas for you:

- **Aerobic Activity**

    Aerobic activity is an effective way to relieve stress because it gets your blood circulating and releases hormones that make you feel better. Try one of these fun activities for the whole family:

    ➤ Biking

    ➤ Hiking or walking

    ➤ Jump roping

> Hula hooping

> Swimming

Do not worry about carving out significant chunks of time for an aerobic workout if you have a busy schedule. Children need 60 minutes of physical activity minimum per day, but this can be divided into smaller chunks.

- **Yoga**

  Yoga is a mix of meditation and exercise that is excellent for cleansing the mind and reducing stress. Yoga, like stretching, can be beneficial in helping your child relax before bed. It is also a good way to start the day with a clear head.

  Here are some stress-relieving yoga poses to be done in a sequence:

  > Stand up with your legs at a hip-width distance and do a swan dive. Hold for a breath while reaching both arms out to your sides and up to the sky. Simultaneously, slowly lower your arms and bend at the waist while maintaining a straight back. Reach for the ground.

  > Place your hands on the ground. Walk backward with your feet until you form an 'A' shape. Look between your hands.

  > Lower your body until you are lying flat on your stomach. Place your palms at a shoulder-width

distance and push your chest up until your back is arching and your stomach muscles are stretched.

> Lower yourself to your stomach once more. Kneel with your knees hip-width apart and push yourself up to your hands and knees. Lower your bottom to your heels by touching your big toes together. Lower your stomach between your knees, rest your forehead on the ground or in your hand, and extend your arms as far as possible. Rest as long as you would like in this position, and repeat the sequence if desired.

- **Stretching**

Stretching can assist you in recognizing and releasing muscle tension. If your child starts to feel stressed throughout the day, teach them to pause and stretch. Stretching before bedtime is also important since it encourages youngsters to relax and prepare for sleep. Here's how to do it:

> Sit with your legs out to the sides; reach for your toes on one side, repeat on the other, and reach down the middle. Hold each posture for 15-30 seconds, keeping your back straight.

> Sit on the ground and touch the bottom side of your feet together before flapping your knees like a butterfly.

7.12 Energize the Mind

Although lack of sleep may not be the core of your child's problems, it can increase stress, intensify anxiety, and have a bad impact on their behavior. Children do not recover as quickly as adults from sleep deprivation.

According to the National Sleep Foundation, kids aged 6 to 13 require 9 to 11 hours of sleep per night.

Furthermore, "falling" asleep is not the same as "going to bed," as a youngster who goes to bed on time may not fall asleep until much later (for a variety of reasons). As a result, quality sleep does not begin until later than parents anticipate.

Establish a regular bedtime routine. Fix a bedtime. Brushing teeth, Bath time, reading, and anything else they do at night should all be done in the same order. This, combined with a consistent bedtime, alerts the body that sleep is approaching. The bedtime routine should conclude in the child's room and be calming.

Finally, keep screen time to an hour or two before bedtime. The brain will be stimulated by noises, bright lights, or loud music. That stimulus makes us feel more awake and aware by slowing our body's natural melatonin production, which helps us fall asleep.

7.13 Incorporate Mindfulness in Routine

Mindfulness means being aware of the present moment, slowing down, and paying attention to what is happening right now. By strengthening connectivity between the prefrontal cortex and the amygdala, mindfulness meditation can improve a patient's ability to regulate emotions and decrease general anxiety disorder symptoms. Furthermore, MRI scans suggest that the amygdala, the brain's "fight or flight" center appears to shrink following an eight-week mindfulness exercise. This primitive brain region, which is linked to fear and emotion, is engaged in initiating the body's stress response. So how can you include it in your child's routine?

- **Mindful Eating**

  Mindful eating is an excellent method to introduce youngsters to the concept of mindfulness. Invite your kid to connect with the experience of eating by noticing what their food looks, smells, and sounds like before they start eating.

  Encourage your child to investigate all of the feelings associated with their food: What is the feeling of having food in your mouth? Is the texture of one food identical to that of another? What about the sweetness or saltiness of the food? Is the flavor of your meal changing as you chew?

  This is a fantastic chance for your youngster to become aware of their body's finely honed senses. Encourage children to recognize some of the cues sent to them by their body and mind, whether hungry or full.

- **Walking Meditation**

  For youngsters, especially those who are new to meditative practices, walking meditation is a fun activity. As you walk down the street with your child, ask them to focus on their feet: How does it feel to have your foot suspended in the air vs. touching the ground? Is it possible for your full foot to touch the ground at once while walking?

  When going from one location to another, you can also encourage your child to use their five senses: In one situation, what do they hear, see, touch, and smell, whereas in another, what do they see, hear, touch, and smell? What emotions are evoked by such features of the physical environment?

- **Think Outside the Box**

  Encourage your youngster to tell you about their day with colors instead of the usual "how was your day?" question at dinner. Colors are pleasant and visual descriptors that youngsters can use to reflect on their experiences because they are strongly related to emotions.

  You're establishing an exploration space for your child to unpack the events that mirror that color by asking them to think about their day differently. This question might also spark a discussion on emotional states and the numerous circumstances that can cause them.

Visualizing emotions as colors might also assist children in understanding that emotional states are fleeting.

Make it a family activity to practice mindfulness. Choose a time during the day when the family can discuss what they did or how they felt during the day. Make this a regular part of the family dinner conversation and include it into the sleep routine. You may even choose a room in the house where you can relax and converse.

7.14 Model Healthy Behavior

We are our children's first teachers as parents. They keep an eye on our actions and see what we do when stressed. We must also set an example of appropriate, healthy coping mechanisms. What are some of your coping mechanisms? – Do you enjoy working out at the gym? Knit? Do you want to do a crossword puzzle?

Share your coping skills with your child the next time you use one. Acknowledge it out loud. "Right now, I am extremely stressed, and all I want is a quick break." For the next fifteen minutes, I am going to knit."

It is also fine if you react overly strongly to a particular stressor on occasion. Simply state how you could have handled the situation better and why you behaved the way you did. Explain why you were frustrated when you were late for work one morning trying to get kids to school and how you could work together to develop better solutions.

Be cautious about how you discuss stress with your child. When expressing your tension, be conscious of who is listening, as children who overhear may begin to worry themselves.

Stress will always linger around your child, but how your child deals with it matters. The earlier your child can learn these healthy coping skills, the more diverse their coping repertoire is.

Conclusion

Children, like adults, experience worry and anxiety from time to time.

Anxiety is a broad term referring to a state of acute worry or unease. It is common to feel uneasy after experiencing something upsetting.

It becomes a problem when anxiety begins to interfere with a child's daily life. A night time ritual performed in homes all around the world involves parents fearlessly pacing the perimeter of bedrooms with a flashlight in hand to show a scared youngster that there are no multi-legged, hairy creatures hiding under their bed. But it becomes a problem when spider phobia keeps you from sleeping away from home or traveling. It is not the spider that keeps the child from trying new things; it is him—and his anxiety—that keeps him from trying new things.

If you walk into any school during test season, you will notice that all of the students are nervous, but some may be so nervous that they do not make it to school that day. This type of severe anxiety can have a negative impact on a child's mental and emotional well-being, as well as their self-esteem and confidence. They may withdraw and go to considerable efforts to avoid situations or things that make them anxious. Anxiety problems in children can be diagnosed in a variety of ways. The specific disorder is determined by what the child is having the most difficulty with, but many of the symptoms are consistent.

According to research, both hereditary and environmental variables contribute to the chance of developing an anxiety disorder. According to studies, biology, biochemistry, life events, and learned habits all have a role.

Anxiety disorders manifest in both physical and psychological manifestations. The age of the child and the kind of anxiety disorder determine how the disorder emerges.

When children are persistently anxious, even the most well-intentioned parents, in their desire to protect their children from harm, can exacerbate the child's worry. It happens when parents want to protect their children from their worries.

This is where this book offers its helping hand. "Anxiety Control for Kids" is an all-in-one solution for your child's anxiety. The book focuses on providing parents with a complete understanding of the problem and then practical strategies to manage it.

The first three chapters of this anxiety book focus on the theoretical part of developing concepts, and the last four chapters include solutions to worry, fear, insecurities, and stress.

The first chapter is devoted to transporting to your child's world of anxiety with real-life stories, so you understand what your child feels. Moving on, it helps you deliver the concept of anxiety to your kids because, at this age, it is particularly hard to understand what they are feeling.

The second chapter explores the causes of our child's anxiety and the part you may unconsciously be playing in growing it, e.g., faster child development, overstuffed schedules, media saturation and adult content, familial changes, teasing & bullying, fewer outlets for stress, parental over shielding and parental avoidance behavior, etc.

The third chapter includes the effects of anxiety on little kids as poor learning and school performance, social withdrawal, sleep disturbances, low self-esteem, panic attacks, unhealthy eating habits, impaired bodily and brain function.

The fourth chapter explains parental strategies for helping your child overcome excessive worry such as connecting with sympathy, creating a worry dump period, validating feelings, distinguishing between real vs. false alarms, changing thought patterns, personifying your child's worry, creating a relaxation kit, and distinguishing between solvable vs. non-solvable worries, etc.

The fifth chapter explains parental strategies for helping your child overcome excessive fear, such as talking about it, filling in the gaps, making a trigger list, regulating scary media consumption, rewiring the memory association, showing relaxation techniques, encouraging realistic thinking, and teaching self-regulation, etc.

The sixth chapter explains parental strategies for helping your child overcome insecurities. These include teaching them self-love, cognitive reframing, developing friendship skills, monitoring their social media, stopping comparing, knowing when to step back, equipping them with knowledge, etc.

The seventh chapter explains parental strategies for helping your child overcome excessive stress such as reframing stress, changing fixed mindset to growth mindset, putting a stop to catastrophic thinking, teaching positive self-talk, stopping overscheduling, teaching problem solving, energizing the body and mind, incorporating mindfulness in routine and model healthy behavior, etc.

I have developed this book with effective strategies as a child psychologist, hoping it helps children worldwide live healthy and happy life. If you found this book helpful, please leave a review on amazon.

Printed in the USA
CPSIA information can be obtained
at www.ICGtesting.com
LVHW022157070924
790454LV00009B/587